Blood and its Diseases

I. Chanarin
M.D., F.R.C.Path.
Consultant Haematologist, Head of Section of Haematology
in the Clinical Research Centre, Northwick Park Hospital.

Milica Brozović
M.D., M.R.C.Path.
Consultant Haematologist, Central Middlesex Hospital.

Elizabeth Tidmarsh
F.I.M.L.S., M.I.Biol.
Chief Medical Laboratory Scientific Officer, Blood Transfusion Laboratory,
Northwick Park Hospital.

D. A. W. Waters
F.I.M.L.S.
Senior Chief Medical Laboratory Scientific Officer, Haematology Department,
Northwick Park Hospital.

SECOND EDITION

CHURCHILL LIVINGSTONE
EDINBURGH LONDON AND NEW YORK 1980

CHURCHILL LIVINGSTONE
Medical Division of the Longman Group Limited

Distributed in the United States of America by
Churchill Livingstone Inc, 19 West 44th Street, New York,
NY 10036, and by associated companies,
branches and representatives throughout
the world.

First Edition 1976
Japanese Edition 1979
Second Edition 1980

ISBN 0 443 02191 0

British Library Cataloguing in Publication Data
Blood and its diseases – 2nd ed
   1. Blood – Diseases
   I. Chanarin, Israel
   616.1'5   RC636   79-42771

Printed in Hong Kong by Wing Tai Cheung Printing Co. Ltd.

Blood and its Diseases

Preface to the Second Edition

The text has been revised, brought up to date and somewhat expanded. References for further reading have been added at the end of each chapter. I hope the book will continue to be of value to those requiring a compact account of the physiology of blood and its disorders.

Harrow, 1980   I. Chanarin

Preface to the First Edition

The intention of this book is to cover the field of haematology in some depth but yet remain both readable and brief. The text is intended to meet the requirements of technicians taking examinations in haematology and doctors taking the examinations of the Royal Colleges of Pathology and Physicians in the UK.

For technicians this book is intended to be complementary to a book devoted to haematological technique. It contains more than will be required for HNC examinations and provides a basis for the advanced examination.

The text should meet the needs of the primary examination in haematology of the Royal College of Pathologists.

The material has been arranged into a section on physiology followed by a consideration of disease states. It is hoped that this arrangement will commend itself to some concerned with undergraduate education. A consideration of physiology in earlier years should be followed by a consideration of the disease states in subsequent years. A full account, for example, of pernicious anaemia, is contained in the section dealing with the physiology of vitamin B_{12} in Chapter 4, followed by the section dealing with megaloblastic anaemia in Chapter 12, and finally with the special features found in pernicious anaemia which are also contained in Chapter 12.

Specialization in haematology is such that no one person can cover the field adequately. I have been fortunate in obtaining the co-operation of my colleagues, Dr Milica Brozović who is responsible for the sections dealing with blood coagulation, Mr D. Waters for the section on laboratory organization and quality control, and Miss Beth Tidmarsh for the section concerned with blood transfusion.

References to original papers have not been included as they are of limited value to those wishing to acquire a broad knowledge of the field. Further selected reading however, is indispensable to those taking the more advanced examinations and a list of recommended books is given.

Finally I wish to acknowledge my indebtedness to Mrs Pat

Goldwater for her careful typing of the manuscript and to Miss C. Allen for the illustrations.

Harrow, 1976   I. Chanarin

Contents

Part 1 PHYSIOLOGY

1

Blood formation and its control

Blood formation (haemopoiesis) normally occurs in the bone marrow which is a mixture of fat and blood-forming cells. The blood supply to the marrow comes via one or more arteries through the outer shell of the bone (cortex), and the vessel ultimately divides into fine thin-walled sinuses. The developing blood cells lie outside the sinuses and mature cells enter the vessels through gaps or by migration between sinus cells. Blood formation is not always confined to marrow. In the unborn child the liver is the principal site of blood formation being full of developing red cells (erythroblasts). This is one of the extra-medullary sites as compared to a marrow (medullary) site of haemopoiesis. With increasing age active blood formation decreases in limb bones, being found only at the tops of the long bones of the limbs and in skull, vertebrae, pelvis and chest bones.

Marrow fragments may be aspirated for examination with a syringe, a special needle (Klima, Salah) being pushed into the marrow through the bony cortex under local anaesthetic. Suitable sites are the tibia in infants, the iliac crest, the sternum or the tips of the vertebral spines.

The stem-cell compartment. Circulating haemopoietic cells develop from a precursor present in very small but relatively constant numbers in the peripheral blood and marrow. This pluripotential and self-maintaining population has been identified by its capacity to repopulate the marrow in induced aplasia. In lethally irradiated mice haemopoietic colonies appear in the spleen when small numbers of marrow cells are injected. Each colony arises from a single stem cell and may consist of erythroid cells, myeloid cells, megakaryocytes or be mixed. These stem cells have been called colony forming units—spleen or CFU–S.

These CFU–S cells give rise to committed stem cells and these may multiply in response to humoral agents, and then differentiate along red, white, lymphoid or megakaryocytic lines. This development has been studied by growing blood colonies in semi-solid media such as plasma clots or methylcellulose, seeded with 'stem' cells derived from marrow or blood.

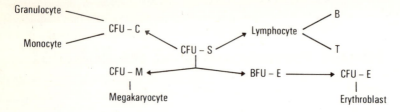

The megakaryocyte and erythroid series may share a common committed stem cell sensitive to erythropoietin and this observation explains the rise in the platelet count in blood loss anaemia when the erythropoietin level increases but a separate 'thrombopoietin' probably occurs and may be present in plasma. CFU–S in the presence of erythropoietin give rise first to burst-forming units—erythroid (BFU–E) which consist of several adjacent colonies of haemoglobin-containing cells, and these develop into colony forming units—erythroid (CFU–E) which are larger single collections of haemoglobin forming cells. With this development there is an increased sensitivity to erythropoietin, the first recognizable cell in this series being a proerythroblast.

Red cell development may involve the co-operation of a helper T-lymphocyte since it has been reported that in its absence erythroid colonies do not develop. Marrow failure may be due to immune reactions directed against erythroid stem cells. Further, a separate population of erythroid precursors responding only to higher levels of erythropoietin produce cells synthesizing fetal haemoglobin and this may be the explanation for the small rise in Hb F levels in some untreated adult anaemias such as pernicious anaemia.

The committed stem cell producing granulocytic colonies called colony forming unit in culture (CFU–C) responds to a humoral factor called colony stimulating factor (CSF) that from human urine being a small molecular weight (45 000) glycoprotein. CSF is also present in leucocytes and monocytes.

The other evidence for a pluripotential stem cell arises from observations on the distribution of an abnormal chromosome, the Philadelphia chromosome, in red, white and megakaryocytic series in chronic myeloid leukaemia. This chromosome is absent in cells of other tissues in this disease and implies a mutation in a stem cell common to these 3 cell lines.

Development from the stem cell. At least two cells can be seen in normal marrow that are not recognizably committed to a particular line of development. One is the so-called *reticulum cell* and the other the *haemocytoblast*. The reticulum cell is very distinctive. It is a large cell, irregular in shape, with abundant cytoplasm containing distinctive pink-staining granules. The nucleus is round with an open lacy chromatin and one or more distinctive, round or oval nucleoli (Fig. 1.1).

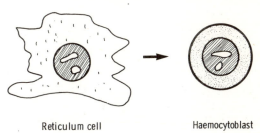

Reticulum cell   Haemocytoblast

Fig. 1.1 Reticulum cell and haemocytoblast.

The haemocytoblast can be seen to be a development from the reticulum cell. The nucleus remains the same but the cytoplasm rounds up and becomes deeply basophilic, that is, staining blue with basic dyes such as methylene blue (Fig. 1.1). Cells with partially basophilic cytoplasmic staining can be seen while the rest of the cytoplasm still shows the pattern of the reticulum cell. The cell in marrow that stores iron is sometimes called a reticulum cell and this is quite different from the cell discussed here.

Red cell formation (erythropoiesis). The earliest cell that can be recognized as belonging to the red cell series is called a *proerythroblast*. It is a large cell with the usual features of an early marrow precursor—a large nucleus with nucleoli and a basophilic cytoplasm. The nucleolus is a paler-staining, sharply-defined, round or oval zone in the nucleus. At this early stage the iron needed for haemoglobin formation is taken into the cell. Thereafter this cell undergoes three, possibly four, mitotic divisions so that each proerythroblast gives rise to eight or 16 cells (Fig. 1.2). The time from proerythroblast to mature red cell is four to six days.

During this development the nucleus gets progressively smaller until it becomes 'pyknotic'. This nucleus is then extruded from the cell. At the same time haemoglobin is synthesized in increasing amount, and the basophilic material (much of it ribosenucleic acid or RNA) is disappearing. Thus the cytoplasm (stained by Romanowsky stains) changes from blue to grey to pink. Concurrently the cell is getting smaller.

With the loss of nucleoli the cell is called a *basophilic* or *early normoblast* (or erythroblast). With the appearance of haemoglobin (a grey cytoplasm), the cell is called a *late* or *polychromatic normoblast*. The late normoblast does not undergo mitosis.

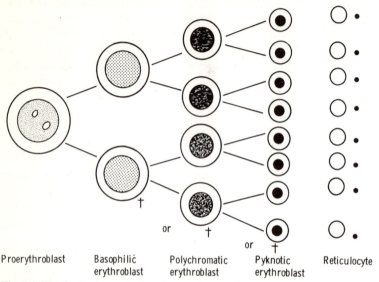

| Proerythroblast | Basophilic erythroblast | Polychromatic erythroblast | Pyknotic erythroblast | Reticulocyte |

Fig. 1.2 The developing red cell undergoes three to four mitotic divisions so that theoretically 8 or 16 cells arise from each proerythroblast. In practice about one cell in eight fails to mature into an erythrocyte. This has been designated as a †.

Finally, after the nucleus is extruded, the red cell is still more basophilic than a mature red cell when stained with Romanowsky stains (eosin-methylene blue mixtures). This grey appearance is called polychromasia and is due to residual RNA in the cytoplasm. At this stage the cell is called a *reticulocyte*. The reticulocyte remains in the marrow for a further one to two days and is then released to the peripheral blood. The reticulocyte loses its basophilia in about 20 hours after being released from the marrow. If blood is mixed with a dye such as brilliant cresyl blue or new methylene blue, the RNA in the reticulocyte gets precipitated as strands in the red cell so that such new blood cells can be counted. They do not constitute more than 2 per cent of normal blood cells. Erythroblasts and reticulocytes in the marrow are 'sticky' and adhere to other marrow cells. With maturation this is lost leading to their release into blood. Normally some 10–15 per cent of developing red cells fail to mature and die in the marrow.

Control of red cell production. Just under one per cent of all red cells are destroyed daily and replaced by new red cells from the marrow.

The fundamental regulatory factor is the amount of oxygen the red cells are able to deliver to the tissues. The red cells passing through the lungs take up oxygen from air, bind this to haemoglobin and release the oxygen in the smallest blood vessels (capillaries), so that it rapidly diffuses out of the red cells, across the capillary wall and into the tissues. Changes in tissue oxygenation result in an appropriate change in red cell production. The best example of this is that people living at high altitude have much higher red cell counts than those at sea level. The partial pressure of oxygen in the inspired air is less at high altitude and less oxygen is taken up by red cells and less gets to the tissues. The response is to increase the amount of oxygen carrier (red cells) to improve delivery of oxygen to tissues.

Oxygen lack in tissues leads to increased release of erythropoietin, a substance which acts directly on the marrow leading to increased cell production. The kidney is believed to be the main site of production of this stimulatory substance producing a 'renal erythropoietic factor' which reacts with plasma to give the active substance. Erythropoietin stimulates stem cells to develop into red cell precursors. It is present in human plasma and the urine and may be assayed by *in vivo* methods using the effects of erythropoietin in stimulating uptake of radioactive iron in mice. The mice are made polycythaemic before the test (to reduce their erythropoietin levels) by injection of blood or by keeping them in a low oxygen-tension chamber.

Another mechanism that may regulate erythropoiesis has been termed 'end-product feedback', that is, products released by red cell destruction themselves influence the rate of red cell production. Haemolytic anaemia where end products of red cell breakdown remain is accompanied by a much more brisk response than anaemia due to blood loss.

White cell production (granulopoiesis). The first recognizable white cell precursor to evolve from the stem cell is a *myeloblast*. Again it is a round cell with a large round nucleus with nucleoli and basophilic cytoplasm. Its differentiation from a proerythroblast is learnt by looking at marrow films rather than by description. This cell undergoes mitotic division and develops into the *promyelocyte* which has pink granules throughout the cytoplasm. These granules contain enzymes such as peroxidase. The promyelocyte also divides and matures (Fig. 1.3). Its maturation is accompanied by loss of nucleoli and appearance of new granules. The cell is now called a *myelocyte*. If the granules are discrete and pink it is a *neutrophil myelocyte*, if the granules are large, deep pink and tear drop in shape it is an *eosinophil myelocyte*, and if the granules are purple to black and tear drop in shape it is a *basophil myelocyte*. The myelocyte can still divide and it matures by changing its round or oval nucleus to a more horseshoe or curved shape. This cell, the *metamyelocyte* does not divide any further but matures into a *polymorphonuclear leucocyte* which may be neutrophil, eosinophil or basophil depending on its granulation. There may be 4 to 5 cell divisions from the myeloblast to the myelocyte stage and the major increase in numbers occurs at the myelocyte level. The period of cell multiplication from myeloblast to myelocyte takes 7–8 days. The period of maturation from metamyelocyte to polymorph takes 6–7 days but this can be shortened to 48 hours in infections.

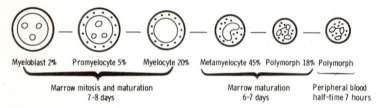

Myeloblast 2%   Promyelocyte 5%   Myelocyte 20%   Metamyelocyte 45%   Polymorph 18%   Polymorph

Marrow mitosis and maturation
7-8 days

Marrow maturation
6-7 days

Peripheral blood
half-time 7 hours

Fig. 1.3 Development of white cells. The change from myeloblast to promyelocyte is accompanied by appearance of granules in the cytoplasm. Transition from promyelocyte to myelocyte is accompanied by the disappearance of nucleoli from the nucleus. The metamyelocyte remains in the marrow for six to seven days before becoming a polymorph.

In a normal marrow developing white cells outnumber normoblasts by two to 20 fold and more than half of these white cells are at the metamyelocyte-polymorph stage. Radioactive phosphorus (^{32}P) given intravenously as sodium phosphate, is incorporated into phosphates in cells and may be used to study granulopoiesis and the appearance of labelled cells in the blood.

In the circulation half the polymorphs adhere to the inside surface of blood vessels (marginating cells), and the other half circulate in the blood and exchange with the marginating pool. Half the polymorphs leave the circulation within six to seven hours and they do so in response to specific needs for such cells in the tissues in a random fashion.

Control of white cell production. Inflammation which is the local response in the body to tissue damage or infection is accompanied by a mobilization of neutrophils to the site. It has been suggested that a 'neutrophil-releasing factor' ultimately mobilizes such cells from marrow and stimulates further production. Factors in human serum and urine (colony-stimulating factor) encourage growth of human marrow granulocytes in agar culture. Possibly this factor may be concerned in control of white cell production.

Monocytes and macrophages. The monocyte developing in the marrow from a more primitive nucleated precursor (monoblast and promonocyte) enters the blood as the familiar monocyte or mononuclear cell and then leaves for the tissues where it is the tissue macrophage. The phagocytic activity of what was once termed the 'reticuloendothelial system' is now becoming equated with the activity of this cell. It appears to share a committed stem cell with other granulocytes since colony culture often yields mixed colonies. The half time of monocytes is blood in 8 hours and like granulocytes they have a circulating and marginating pool.

If the tissue macrophage is the blood monocyte which has migrated to the tissues then it clearly has properties that differentiate it from other mature granulocytes. It is capable of cell division and of fusing with other macrophages to form multinucleate giant cells.

Lymphocytes. These arise from lymphoblasts in marrow and further replication occurs in lymph follicles of lymph glands situated throughout the body.

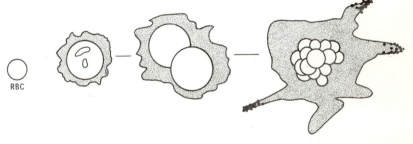

RBC

Young megakaryocyte   Mature megakaryocyte

Fig. 1.4 Megakaryocyte nuclei continue to divide until 8–16 are present in a mature cell. Platelets are shed from the periphery of the cell.

Platelet production. The parent cell in the marrow, the megakaryocyte, arises from a stem cell. The earliest form is a very large cell with a diameter three times that of a red cell. It has a large round nucleus, prominent nucleoli and a thin rim of cytoplasm that characteristically has a very irregular edge (Fig. 1.4). The nucleus continues to divide until the mature megakaryocyte has 8–16 nuclei. The time from stem cell to platelet-producing cell is about 10 days. Platelets form in the cytoplasm and are often seen as strings of platelets coming from the edges of the cell. In a normal marrow active platelet budding may be seen on between 20 per cent up to 80 per cent of megakaryocytes. It is said that a megakaryocyte releases about 4000 platelets and thereafter the senescent cell is phagocytosed by macrophages.

A specific humoral regulator of thrombopoiesis exists called thrombopoietin. Fresh plasma infused to a thrombocytopenic child was followed regularly by a substantial but short lived rise in platelet count and it was suggested that the effects were due to the infusion of thrombopoietin.

References

Cline M J 1977 Cellular kinetics of monocytes and macrophages. In: Williams W J, Beutler E, Erslev A J, Rundles R W (eds) Hematology McGraw-Hill, New York. 2nd edn p 869–874

Golde D W, Cline M J 1977 Granulocyte kinetics. In: Williams W J, Beutler E, Erslev A J, Rundles R W (eds) Hematology McGraw-Hill, New York. 2nd edn p 699–706

Lajtha L G 1975 Haemopoietic stem cells. British Journal of Haematology 29: 529–535

Nienhuis A W, Benz J B Jr 1977 Regulation of haemoglobin synthesis during the development of the red cell. New England Journal of Medicine 297: 1318–1328, 1371–1381 and 1430–1436

2

Blood volume, life span and demise of cellular elements of the blood, normal values and normal functions

How much blood?

An estimate of blood volume for normal subjects in relation to height and weight can be obtained from Tables. However, normal people differ considerably in the amount of fat in the body and since fat, as a tissue, holds relatively little blood, variation in the amount of fat can cause considerable error. In clinical practice, that is, where an abnormal result is possible, it is necessary to measure blood volume in each patient.

Red-cell volume. Normal males have 29 ml of red cells for each kg of body weight, and women 25 ml of red cells/kg body weight. These values hold good for normal infants and children. A 70 kg man has 2·1 litres of red cells and woman 1·7 litres. The range is as follows:

```
RBC volume—men     —26-33 ml/kg
           women—22-29 ml/kg
Plasma volume      —35-45 ml/kg
```

Measurement is made by taking a blood sample, incubating the blood with radioactive sodium chromate (^{51}Cr) and reinjecting a measured volume of these labelled red cells into the subject. Mixing of these red cells is normally complete after three minutes. By noting the dilution of the labelled red cells in the subjects circulation, a reliable estimate of the red-cell volume is made. A true whole body PCV is required for the calculation.

Plasma volume. The dilution in plasma of an injected marker substance is used to measure plasma volume. Such a marker must be retained within the plasma compartment after mixing, not pass out to fluid in tissues (extravascular fluids) and not enter cells. In practice human albumin labelled with radioactive iodine or, rarely today, labelled with a blue dye (Evans blue, T-1824) which binds to albumen, is used. Loss of the marker from the circulation leads to overestimation of plasma volume. Red-cell volume and plasma volume should be estimated together with ^{51}Cr-labelled red cells injected first, followed after 10 minutes by an injection of ^{125}I-labelled albumin.

The average normal plasma volume is 39 ml/kg. Thus a 70 kg subject has 2·7 litres of plasma. This would give a normal total blood volume in a 70 kg male of 4·8 litres and female 4·5 litres.

Packed cell volume (PCV or haematocrit)

When a blood sample is placed in a narrow tube and centrifuged the red cells are deposited to occupy about 40 per cent of the blood column, the remaining 60 per cent being occupied by clear plasma. White cells and platelets are deposited on top of the red cell column and reticulocytes tend to form a darker band at the top of the red cell column below the white cells. Under standard condition of centrifugation, the PCV is highly reproducible and this has led to a belief that it is a very reliable index of red cell mass. There are a number of inherent problems in the PCV.

Venous and body haematocrit. If the ratio of plasma to red cells was constant the PCV would give the same answer with blood taken from any site in the body and PCV would be the same as

$$\frac{\text{red cell volume}}{\text{total blood volume}} = \text{body haematocrit}$$

In fact the amount of plasma that moves round with red cells varies in different parts of the body. In small blood vessels plasma moves relatively slowly around the walls and red cells with plasma forms a faster stream in the centre. Thus there is relatively more plasma in small vessels as compared to large ones, so that the PCV in the periphery is lower and this includes organs such as the liver. The ratio of

$$\frac{\text{whole body haematocrit}}{\text{venous haematocrit}}$$

is generally taken as 0·91. This means that when the PCV for venous blood is 40 per cent the whole body haematocrit is 36·4 per cent.

Trapped plasma. It is not possible to pack red cells absolutely by centrifugation. Some plasma is trapped between the red cells. With normal blood under the usual laboratory conditions, some 2·7 per cent of the red-cell column is due to contained plasma.

Effect of posture and stasis. The venous PCV is higher in subjects standing up and lower lying down. There is a loss of plasma after standing up. The change in the PCV (as well as red cell count and haemoglobin) can be about 5 per cent. Pressure of a tourniquet on the arm for longer than one minute also produces a rise in the PCV.

Electronic derivation of the PCV. If the number of red cells is known and their size, the PCV can be calculated. This is done in some automatic blood-counting machines and has the advantage that trapped plasma can be excluded. Under these circumstances normal values for the PCV given as the mean ±2 S.D. are:

Men	42·8±4·9%
Women	39·5±3·7%

Haemoglobin concentration and red cell count

The normal haemoglobin concentration and red cell count as sea level is:

	Men	Women
Haemoglobin g/100 ml	14·7±1·8	13·5±1·2
Red cell count $10^6/\mu l$	5·0±0·6	4·6±0·5

Up to puberty there is no sex difference but thereafter men have higher values. The newborn have higher values with a mean haemoglobin concentration of 17 g/100 ml. This value falls quite rapidly in the first 8–10 weeks of life, largely due to underproduction by the marrow. The haemoglobin continues to fall to about 11 g between 1–2 years of age, and then slowly rises to about 12·5 g in the 3–6 year age period.

Altitude has a major influence on normal blood values. People normally living at 14 900 ft above sea level have an average red-cell volume of 64 ml/kg and a plasma volume of 36 ml/kg. The haemoglobin concentration is 20·8 g/100 ml and red-cell count 6·1 million/μl. At an altitude of 4000 feet above sea level the mean haemoglobin in man is 16·9 g/100 ml.

Absolute values

The size of the red cell, its haemoglobin content and haemoglobin concentration can be calculated from the red cell count, haemoglobin concentration and PCV.

$$\text{Mean Corpuscular volume (MCV)} = \frac{PCV \times 10}{RBC} \text{ fl}$$

$$\text{Mean Corpuscular haemoglobin (MCH)} = \frac{Hb}{RBC \times 100\,000} \text{ pg}$$

$$\text{Mean Corpuscular haemoglobin concentration (MCHC)} = \frac{Hb \times 100}{PCV} \text{ \%}$$

These values depend not only on the accuracy with which the data are estimated, but also on whether the PCV includes trapped plasma or not. The effect of trapped plasma is to give a falsely high value for the PCV and hence too high a value for the MCV, and too low a value for the MCHC.

Older texts give the range for the MCV as 75–96 fl. When trapped plasma is excluded the range is healthy normal controls is 80–90 fl. The changes in the MCV in the first few years of life are shown in figure 2.1. The macrocytosis of the newborn is replaced by microcytosis between 1–2 years of age. The normal MCH ranges from 27–32 pg (mean 29·3), and the normal MCHC from 32–36 per cent.

Erythrocyte sedimentation rate (ESR)
When blood is diluted in isotonic citrate (four parts blood to one part citrate) and the red cells allowed to settle in a vertical 200 mm tube (Westergren tube) at room temperature, the length of clear plasma at the top is 0–5 mm after an hour in men, and up to 7 mm per hour in women. The rate of fall of red cells is determined by the tendency to rouleaux formation. Rouleaux refers to the tendency of red cells to adhere together to resemble stacks of coins. The larger clumps of red cells fall more rapidly. The amount of rouleaux formed is determined by the concentration of proteins in plasma, the most important being fibrinogen and less important, globulins and glycoproteins. Blood collected into EDTA and subsequently diluted in citrate has the same ESR as a specimen collected directly into citrate.

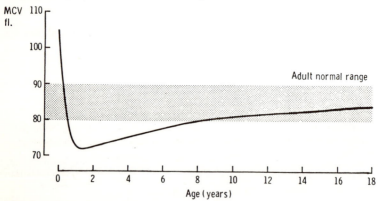

Fig. 2.1 The red blood cells in the newborn are macrocytic. Over the next few months this is replaced by microcytosis, adult values being attained only in the second decade.

An abnormally raised ESR is used as a non-specific screen for ill health and as a means of checking the activity of chronic diseases such as tuberculosis. Nevertheless, disease can be present with a normal

ESR. The ESR is more rapid after the age of 60, values of up to 20 mm in an hour being found.

Plasma viscosity may be used instead of the ESR and has a similar significance.

Life span of red blood cells
The normal red cell survives in the normal circulation for about 110 days. The life span may be measured in two ways.

Cohort label. Here a label is incorporated into the developing cell in the marrow. Such a label is any substance that is normally incorporated into red cells. Thus ^{15}N-glycine is used to make the haem of haemoglobin. ^{75}Selenomethionine can take the place of methionine in protein molecules such as globin. ^{59}Fe can be incorporated into the haem of the haemoglobin molecule. Giving of any of these materials leads to labelling of a single generation or cohort of red cells. The label will then disappear from the blood at the end of the life of those cells, and a labelled end product may be excreted. The pattern is shown in figure 2.2.

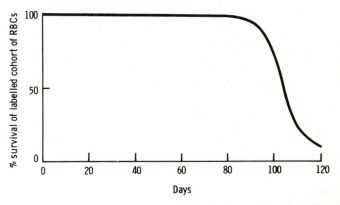

Fig. 2.2 A cohort label labels a single generation of new red blood cells. The label will be retained in the red cells until the death of these cells about 110 days later.

Random label. An aliquot of the subjects red cells is incubated with either ^{51}Cr or DF^{32}P. The label binds to either the haemoglobin in the case of chromium or other cell component, and when returned to the circulation the survival of the labelled red cells may be followed. Here the label is attached to red cells of different ages some of which may be nearing the end of their life span, others may be relatively young. A regular amount of these red cells will disappear from the circulation daily. The pattern of survival is illustrated in figure 2.3.

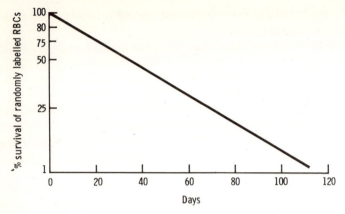

Fig. 2.3 A random label like ⁵¹Cr, labels red cells of different ages. These disappear from the circulation according to their age, the old ones first etc. Thus there is a steady disappearance of the label from blood. Theoretically the label should finally disappear when the youngest cells come to the end of their life (about 110 days later). In practice because of elution of the label (⁵¹Cr) from the red cells the slope is much steeper.

Ashby method. The survival of transfused donor cells can be followed for example, when group O blood is given to a group A recipient. The group A cells can be removed from samples by agglutination with an anti-A serum and the remaining free (un-agglutinated) O cells counted.

Demise of blood cells and the spleen

Some data are available about the disposal of abnormal red cells which have a reduced mean cell life span but virtually none about how normal but senescent red cells are dealt with. Nor do we know the features that distinguish such a senescent red blood cell. It seems probable however that the same mechanisms operate under both circumstances. Abnormal red blood cells are removed by the spleen particularly when the defect is relatively mild, such as a small amount of anti-D on a rhesus-positive cell. More severely abnormal red cells, for example with a large dose of anti-D, are cleared by both liver and spleen. Markedly defective red cells undergo intravascular haemolysis in the circulation. Within the spleen and liver the cells are phagocytosed by tissue macrophages.

It is probable that the spleen plays a role in the removal of old red cells although it should be added that splenectomy does not produce any detectable changes in this process other than persistence of particular cells that would normally be culled by the spleen such as those with Howell-Jolly bodies, etc. The structure of the spleen is such that slow passage of red cells occurs in a macrophage-rich environment. The arteries in the trabeculae of the spleen instead of narrowing to arterioles, capillaries and joining the venous system, end abruptly so that the arterial blood empties into spaces called splenic cords. This blood then passes into splenic sinusoids which join veins. The central arteries in addition have other arteries leading off at right angles to the main artery so that plasma at the margin of the artery can pass into these vessels leaving red cells in the axial stream to pass on. The two main cells in the spleen are small lymphocytes and tissue macrophages and these surround the central arteries forming the white pulp. Between the areas of white pulp is the red pulp. This consists of sinuses and splenic cords filled with red cells. The sinuses are made up of flat endothelial cells and some red cells make their way through these endothelial cells. The openings in this discontinuous membrane are about 3 μm in size. Red cells that lack deformability whether due to spherocytosis, sickled haemoglobin, precipitated globin (Heinz bodies), or containing malarial parasites will fail to pass these openings and allow macrophages to engulf all or part of the cell. As indicated the changes in otherwise normal but old red cells that lead to their removal are undetermined.

White blood cells
Normal values are:

Total WBC count	4000–11 000/μl
Neutrophils	2000–7500/μl
Lymphocytes	1500–3500/μl
Monocytes	200–800/μl
Eosinophils	40–440/μl
Basophils	0–100/μl

The total white cell count in the newborn can be as high as 40 000/μl and values up to 24 000/μl may be normal throughout the first six months of life. Thereafter values up to 13 000/μl may be encountered normally and adult ranges are reached after the age of 18. The higher white cell count in childhood is due to a higher lymphocyte count, the other cells being present in the same number as in adults after the first year of life.

Platelets
The normal platelet count is 100–400 × 10^9/l. When platelets are labelled with ^{51}Cr and given to healthy individuals, about two thirds

remain in the plasma. The remaining one third is pooled in the spleen, from which it is exchanged freely but slowly with the plasma pool. In patients with an enlarged spleen 80–90 per cent of the platelets may be sequestered in the spleen.

Human platelets labelled with ^{51}Cr, DF^{32}P, ^{119}In or aspirin have a life span of 8 to 12 days. It is still uncertain whether platelet destruction is random or due to senescence. The sites of platelet destruction are liver and spleen; in autoradiographic studies following transfusion of isotopically-labelled platelets, the isotopes were also found in endothelial cells, but the magnitude of endothelial–platelet interaction is undertermined.

Functions of blood

Blood is concerned with the transport of gases, with the transport of materials for the provision of energy and for synthesis, with transport of substances concerned with defence against foreign organisms, with overcoming the effects of injury and with the transport of substances regulating the body's activities (hormones).

Red cells. These function in the transfer of oxygen from lungs to tissues and in the return of carbon dioxide to the lungs. The special features within the red cell and in the haemoglobin molecule that enable the red cell to perform these functions efficiently are discussed in chapters 3 and 5.

Neutrophil polymorphs. The prime function of these cells is to engulf (phagocytose) and breakdown a variety of substances including bacteria. Neutrophils move rapidly to areas of injury or infection. Local events alter the permeability of small blood vessels so that neutrophils migrate out from their marginating position in the vessels into the tissues and are attracted to the site of insult by production of humoral substances (Fig. 2.4). This process is *chemotaxis.* Some of the components of complement (a number of protein and enzymatic substances in plasma concerned with immune reactions) play a role in chemotaxis.

Having arrived at the site, the neutrophil comes into surface contact with the foreign substance and ingests it (pinocytosis). This process is aided by specific antibody and complement (these were once called opsonins). These processes require active energy provided by anaerobic glycolysis (see Ch. 5).

Within the cell the bacteria are killed and digested. Lysosomal granules empty their contents into the phagocytic vacuole so that hydrolytic enzymes are able to act on the ingested particle. Hydrogen peroxide H_2O_2), a powerful oxidizing substance is produced possibly via the pentose–phosphate shunt (Ch. 5), and is of prime importance in bacterial killing. Lysozyme, an enzyme splitting amino-sugars, is also produced but is probably of minor importance. Such neutrophils now reduce the dye nitroblue tetrazolium (NBT) a reaction that is sometimes useful in detecting infection. H_2O_2 is removed by the enzyme catalase. Neutrophil granules contain an enzyme myelo-peroxidase which also attacks bacteria. Some bacteria however, such as *M. tuberculosis* and *Brucella* are resistant to destruction by neutrophils.

Eosinophil polymorphs. Their function is not known. They increase in number in blood and tissues in worm (helminth) infestation, and in allergic diseases such as asthma and hay fever. They are also capable of phagocytosis in the same way as described for the neutrophil.

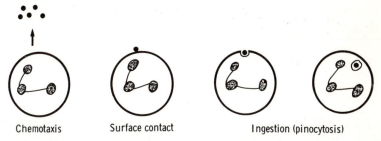

Chemotaxis   Surface contact   Ingestion (pinocytosis)

Fig. 2.4 The sequence by which a polymorph engulfs an organism involves attraction to the organism (chemotaxis) and ingestion (pinocytosis). Thereafter the organism is digested by hydrolytic enzymes.

Basophil polymorphs. The granules of these cells contain histamine and heparin. The tissue counterpart is the mast cell. The basophil appears to play a role in acute hypersensitivity and allergic reactions, these being mediated at the end organ through histamine release. Many of these reactions are antibody mediated involving IgE immunoglobulins on the cell surface.

Monocytes. This cell in the tissues is referred to as a macrophage. It migrates to areas of inflammation and ingests bacteria and particles by the same mechanism that has been described in relation to the neutrophil. It plays an important part in the primary immunological response to an antigen and is believed to process the antigen into a form that the lymphocyte can accept. The macrophages also release or secrete a variety of enzymes that are concerned with the inflammatory response and the disposal of foreign or dead material in tissues.

Lymphocytes. These are the cells that ultimately produce antibody, that initiate an immune response and carry the memory of previous exposure to antigen. This is discussed in chapter 7.

Platelets. Platelets are vital in preventing rupture of small vessels by plugging breaches in the inner endothelial surface. They provide coagulation factors for various stages of the coagulation sequence and ultimately for clot retraction (see Ch. 6).

Plasma. Apart from being the medium in which the red cells, white cells and platelets circulate, plasma contains the coagulation factors required for normal haemostasis and the precursor forms of fibrinolytic enzymes which will remove excess fibrin deposition.

Plasma is the vehicle by which protein products, carbohydrates, fat, iron, vitamins and trace elements pass from gut to liver to tissues. End products of cell activity are taken by plasma for excretion by the kidney, lungs, and biliary tract.

Secretion from endocrine glands (pancreas, thyroid, adrenal, pituitary) are carried by plasma as are antibodies produced as a result of exposure to many infectious agents.

References

Stemerman M B 1974 Platelet interaction with intimal connective tissue. In: Baldini M G, Ebbe S (eds) Platelets; production, function, transfusion and storage. Grune and Stratton, New York, p 157–170

Williams W J, Beutler E, Erslev A J, Rundles R W (eds) 1977 Hematology, 2nd edn, McGraw-Hill, New York

3

Haemoglobin—synthesis, breakdown and function

Haemoglobin is the all important red pigment within the red blood cell. Its prime function is the uptake and delivery of oxygen. An enormous amount of detailed information is known about its formation, structure and function.

An adult has about 630 g of haemoglobin containing about 2·2 g of iron. One per cent is renewed each 24 hours, that is, some 6·3 g of haemoglobin requiring 22 mg of iron are made daily. Each gram of haemoglobin carries 1·34 ml of oxygen. The MW of haemoglobin is 64 500.

Haemoglobin concentration is measured by the absorption of a solution of haemoglobin that has been allowed to react with potassium cyanide and potassium ferricyanide ('Drabkin's Reagent') to form cyanmethaemoglobin. Such a solution has a standard absorption in a spectrophotometer at a wave length of 540 nm. Other methods of standardization have involved measurement of iron content and oxygen-carrying capacity.

Haemoglobin consists of two major portions—the iron-containing haem (or heme) and the protein portion, globin.

Haem
Haem is made up of ringed structures called pyrrole rings (Fig. 3.1). The building materials used to synthesize haem within the developing red cell are the amino acid, glycine, and succinic acid. One molecule of glycine and one of succinate condense to give delta-aminolaevulinic acid—shorted to ALA (Fig. 3.2). Next, two molecules of ALA condense together to give a pyrrole ring. The enzyme bringing about the linkage of two ALA molecules is called δ-aminolaevulinic acid dehydrase (ALA dehydrase). Four pyrrole rings then react to form a tetrapyrrolle ring. The four rings are joined together by carbon atoms (=CH-, methene bridges). This ring is then called a protoporphyrin ring and it has additional structures (with 1, 2 or 3-carbon chains) on the pyrrole rings. At this stage iron is taken up (Fig. 3.3).

All the enzymes carrying out these reactions are present in mitochondria in normoblasts and this is the site of haem synthesis. Mature red cells no longer have mitochondria and hence cannot make haem, nor incorporate iron into haemoglobin. The reticulocyte can still do so. More than 300 mg of haem are made each 24 hours, primarily for

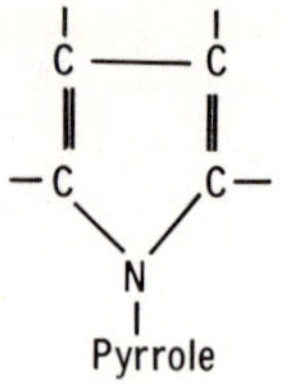

$$
\begin{array}{ccc}
| & & | \\
C & \!\!\!\!-\!\!\!\! & C \\
\| & & \| \\
-C & & C- \\
& N & \\
& | &
\end{array}
$$

Pyrrole

Fig. 3.1 The pyrrole ring.

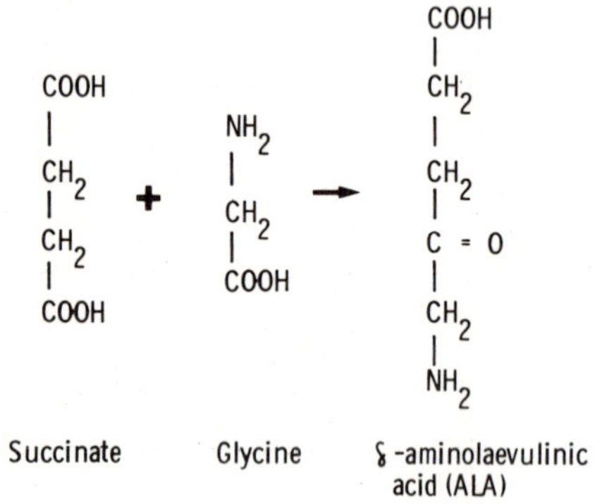

$$
\begin{array}{c}
COOH \\
| \\
CH_2 \\
| \\
CH_2 \\
| \\
COOH
\end{array}
\;+\;
\begin{array}{c}
NH_2 \\
| \\
CH_2 \\
| \\
COOH
\end{array}
\;\longrightarrow\;
\begin{array}{c}
COOH \\
| \\
CH_2 \\
| \\
CH_2 \\
| \\
C = O \\
| \\
CH_2 \\
| \\
NH_2
\end{array}
$$

Succinate   Glycine   δ -aminolaevulinic
                                acid (ALA)

Fig. 3.2 The condensation of succinate and glycine to form δ-aminolaevulinic acid (ALA). Two molecules of ALA condense together to form haem.

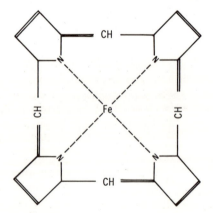

Fig. 3.3 The structure of haem.

haemoglobin but also for myoglobin, cytochrome and catalase, particularly in the liver, all this accounting for about 15 per cent of total haem production.

Globin

This protein is the other major component of haemoglobin. Some 8 g of globin are made daily.

Synthesis. Like all proteins, globin is made up of a long chain of aminoacids, the basic NH_2 group of the one aminoacid being linked to an acidic COOH group of the succeeding aminoacid in peptide or CO:NH bonds. Globin is synthesized on particles in the cell cytoplasm called ribosomes. The basic information on the sequence of aminoacids in the globin chain is held in the normoblast nucleus on the DNA of the gene. This information in turn is passed on to the cytoplasm by the production of a nucleic acid chain that mirrors the DNA chain. This is messenger RNA. The ribosomes move to messenger RNA and the appropriate aminoacid is brought along by a transfer RNA specific for each aminoacid (Fig. 3.4). The aminoacid is attached to the ribosome which moves along messenger RNA when a further aminoacid is attached. In this way a chain of aminoacids in predetermined sequence is formed. When the chain length is complete it drops off the ribosome and associates with another chain to form a dimer ($\alpha\beta$, $\alpha\gamma$, or $\alpha\delta$).

Types. Normal haemoglobin contains four types of globin molecules (monomers or polypeptide chains). These associate together

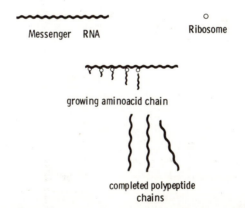

Messenger RNA

Ribosome

growing aminoacid chain

completed polypeptide chains

Fig. 3.4 Messenger RNA carries the coding for the sequence of aminoacids required to build globin. A ribosome moves to m-RNA and the appropriate aminoacid (on the specific transfer RNA) is brought. Further aminoacids are joined on to form the polypeptide globin chain.

first in pairs (dimers) and then in groups of four (tetramers). Each tetramer has two α (alpha) chains, each of which is a sequence of 141 aminoacids. In adult haemoglobin (HbA) 2α chains associate with 2β (beta) chains (146 aminoacids). Two α chains are also associated with 2γ (gamma) chains to give fetal haemoglobin (HbF) and with 2δ (delta) chains to give haemoglobin A_2. Thus the haemoglobin in a normal red cell is as follows:

Haemoglobin A — Hb A — $\alpha_2\beta_2$ 96–98%
Haemoglobin F — Hb F — $\alpha_2\gamma_2$ 0–1%
Haemoglobin A_2 — Hb A_2 — $\alpha_2\delta_2$ 1.5–3%

Configuration. Each globin chain is coiled on itself to form a spheroidal molecule (Fig. 3.5) so that aminoacids which have acidic or basic (polar) groups are directed outwards and neutral (nonpolar) aminoacids are towards the centre of the molecule. Segments of the aminoacid chain are numbered A to H, each segment (or helix) being separated by a bend in the chain. Haem is attached to globin within such a bend in the chain between the E and F helices the link being to a histidine in each helix. The correct link to haem is essential for stability of the chain and failure leads to unfolding of the globin chain and an unstable haemoglobin. As each haemoglobin has four globin chains it has four haem groups each with its atom of iron.

Genetics. In the fetus more than 95 per cent of the haemoglobin is HbF. About four weeks before birth (36 week fetus) HbA begins to

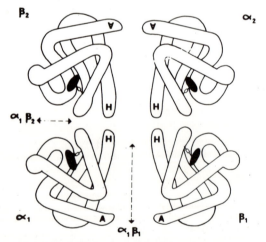

Fig. 3.5 The arrangement of the 4 polypeptide chains of haemoglobin. (Reproduced by courtesy of Professor J. M. White).

increase till at birth HbF is 70–80 per cent and HbA is 20–30 per cent. HbA increases steadily to reach adult level at five months of age. The very young fetus up to 10 weeks of intrauterine life has a different globin chain, termed epsilon ϵ giving a still different haemoglobin. The synthesis of each polypeptide chain is controlled by one or more genetic loci. Thus each normal individual has one locus for β and δ on each of two chromosomes (one from each parent). There may be two loci for control of α chain synthesis and this is based on varying manifestations of disease involving the α chain. There appear to be four loci for control of γ chain synthesis.

Measurement. Production of polypeptide chains is measured by incubating whole blood with a labelled aminoacid such as ^{3}H-leucine. The reticulocytes will take up the aminoacid and incorporate it into globin. A haemolysate is prepared, globin precipitated with acetone and the monomers separated from each other by the addition of a strong solution of urea. The α and β chains are then separated by column chromatography and the radioactivity in the positions of the α and β chains counted. Normally the ratio of these counts is 1·0 indicating that an equal amount of α and other chains are made.

The relative amounts of HbA and A_2 in the red cell are measured by electrophoresis of an haemolysate and elution of the haemoglobin bands. The amount of HbF is measured by taking into account its greater resistance to denaturation at extremes of pH as compared to HbA which is more readily damaged. Thus Singer's method measures the haemoglobin that is left after exposing a haemolysate to alkali for 60 seconds. Similarly, exposure of the red cells on a blood film to pH 3·3 will denature HbA but not HbF, and thus fetal cells (containing mostly HbF) can be detected.

Oxygen transport by haemoglobin

Each 100 ml of arterial (oxygenated) blood carries 19 ml of oxygen in combination with haemoglobin and about 0·3 ml of oxygen in solution in the plasma. The pressure or tension of oxygen in the air in the lungs is equivalent to 100 mm mercury (mmHg). At this tension oxygen passes from lungs to the blood until the arterial blood becomes about 97 per cent saturated with oxygen. When the arterial blood reaches the capillaries in the tissues of the body, it encounters a much lower oxygen tension which is about 40 mmHg. At this lower tissue oxygen tension oxygen will move rapidly from plasma to tissues across the capillary wall, and this is accompanied by rapid shift of oxygen in turn from haemoglobin out of the red cell to plasma and so to the tissues. In the capillaries the oxygen saturation of blood falls to about 70 per cent corresponding to an oxygen content of about 14 ml/100 ml. Some 5 ml of oxygen has been given up to tissues by each 100 ml of blood.

The manner in which oxygen is taken up and released by blood is shown by the oxygen dissociation curve (Fig. 3.6). This may be constructed by exposing blood to known oxygen tensions in a chamber called a tonometer, and when equilibrium has been reached the oxygen carried by the blood is measured either in a Van Slyke apparatus or spectrophotometrically. The shape of the curve illustrates how well adapted is the red cell to transporting oxygen, becoming completely saturated at the oxygen tension in the lung (97 per cent saturated at an

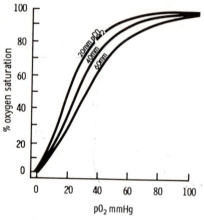

Fig. 3.6 Oxygen dissociation curve and the effect of varying CO_2 tension in changing pH.

oxygen tension of 100 mmHg) and falling to 70 per cent saturation at the lower oxygen tension of tissues (40 mmHg). If the curve shifts to the left, less oxygen is given up at a given oxygen tension. If it shifts to the right, more oxygen is given up at a given tension. The shape of the oxygen dissociation curve may be altered by changes in pH, ionic strength or temperature. More oxygen is given up at a more rapid rate when the acidity and temperature of the blood are increased.

Blood also takes up carbon dioxide (CO_2) which is at a relatively high tension in tissues. Most of this CO_2 passes into the red blood cells where it is converted to carbonic acid (H_2CO_3) by the enzyme carbonic anhydrase. The hydrogen ion released by this weak acid in the red cell is mopped up by haemoglobin itself. Some CO_2 also combines directly with haemoglobin to form carbaminohaemoglobin

$$CO_2 + HbNH \rightleftharpoons HbNHCOOH$$

This uptake of CO_2 and increase in hydrogen ion concentration shifts the oxygen dissociation curve to the right so that more O_2 is given up.

In the lungs the CO_2 tension is lower so that CO_2 is given up. This shifts the oxygen dissociation curve to the left favouring the uptake of oxygen. The effect of pH in altering the dissociation curve is termed the *Bohr effect*.

The ferrous iron in haem has one bond linked to each of four pyrrole groups, a fifth valency (bond) is attached to globin and the sixth valency carries oxygen (O_2). Each haemoglobin molecule has four haem groups, four iron atoms and hence has four oxygen molecules. The oxygen molecules probably get into the haemoglobin molecule one at a time. Once one or more oxygens have linked to the ferrous iron, the remaining haem groups develop an increased affinity for oxygen, the affinity of the haemoglobin for the last O_2 molecule being 20-fold greater than for the first. This effect is called the *haem-haem interaction*. It is due to a change in configuration within the molecule so that there is an outward displacement of the β-globin chains opening up the pocket holding the oxygen molecules.

In addition to the Bohr effect and the haem-haem interaction, the shape of the dissociation curve is influenced by one of the products of glucose breakdown in the cell, *2, 3 disphosphoglycerate* (2,3DPG). The addition of 2,3DPG to haemoglobin reduces its affinity for oxygen, that is, the dissociation curve is shifted to the right. It does so by binding largely to reduced or deoxyhaemoglobin. By lowering oxygen affinity, 2,3DPG tends to make oxygen available more readily to tissues. 2,3DPG does not attach to HbF, and the oxygen dissociation curve of HbF is shifted to the left of that of HbA.

In clinical practice it may be necessary to know arterial oxygen saturation and the affinity of haemoglobin for oxygen. Oxygen saturation of arterial blood is normally over 95 per cent and the pO_2 of arterial blood (partial pressure of oxygen) is over 70 mmHg. Oxygen affinity is the measure of the readiness with which the haemoglobin binds oxygen. It can be measured by constructing an oxygen dissociation curve (when a shift to the left means increased affinity and a shift to the right decreased affinity). More simply the tension of oxygen (pO_2) required to half saturate the haemoglobin (50 per cent saturation) is measured. This is normally about 26–28 mmHg, that is, PO_{50} is normally 26–28 mmHg (see oxygen dissociation curve).

Breakdown of haemoglobin

Old red cells are largely taken up by macrophages in the spleen. The red cells are presumably broken up and the haemoglobin is degraded

in these cells. The haem is split from globin. The globin is broken
down and the aminoacids re-utilized. The haem ring is opened up and
the iron is retained and re-utilized for new haemoglobin synthesis.
Most of the 22 mg iron needed daily comes from this source and only
1–1½ mg from absorption of dietary iron.

With the opening up of the haem ring one of the methene
carbon bridges between the pyrrole rings is converted to carbon
monoxide. This is excreted via the lungs and exhaled carbon monoxide
is a measure of haemoglobin breakdown. The more red cells are broken
down the more carbon monoxide is exhaled so that exhaled carbon
monoxide can be a measure of red cell survival.

The haem is converted to bilirubin (Fig. 3.7). This yellow pigment
is carried to the liver bound to albumin. This compound gives an
indirect reaction in Van den Bergh's test used to measure bilirubin. In
the liver glucuronic acid is attached to bilirubin by an enzyme,
glucuronyl transferase. This process is called conjugation. The
bilirubin is now called conjugated bilirubin and gives a direct Van den

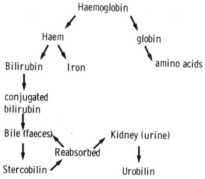

Fig. 3.7 The breakdown of haemoglobin.

Bergh reaction. It is excreted into the bile and hence into the small gut.
In the gut bilirubin is converted to stercobilin. Some stercobilin is reabsorbed into the plasma and re-excreted by the kidney. In the urine it
is called urobilin.

Salvage of haemoglobin iron

The conservation of iron from haem is so important that there are
special mechanisms designed to prevent loss of haem and hence of
iron. Although the breakdown of red cells normally is largely
intracellular, any destruction of red cells in the circulation may release
haemoglobin. The MW of haemoglobin (64 500) is such that if it were

free in plasma it would be excreted by the kidney.

Plasma has a protein (an alpha-globulin) whose function it is to capture or bind free haemoglobin. It is called haptoglobin. There are indeed several types of haptoglobin that differ in their electrophoretic mobility. Each 100 ml of plasma has enough haptoglobin to bind about 100 to 140 mg of haemoglobin. The haemoglobin-haptoglobin complex is large enough not to be excreted by the kidney and it is then taken up by the reticuloendothelial system at a rate of about 15 mg haemoglobin per 100 ml plasma per hour. Haptoglobin is detected by adding free haemoglobin in measured amounts to plasma and noting the position of the haemoglobin-stained band in the α-globulin region on electrophoresis. Once all the haptoglobin has been bound or if none is there, excess haemoglobin will be found in the β-globulin region.

A second protein that binds free haem is called haemopexin and will bind haem when the haptoglobin mechanism is saturated. Haem bound to albumin is transferred to haemopexin. When these mechanisms are saturated free haemoglobin will be excreted into the urine. Hepatic macrophages also take up haemoglobin directly, degrade this to haem which is released from the cell bound to albumin. This compound, methaemalbumen gives a positive Schumm's test, and this is taken as evidence of recent release of haemoglobin in plasma.

References
Weatherall D J, Clegg J B 1972 The Thalassaemia Syndromes. Blackwell, Oxford.

4

Iron, vitamin B$_{12}$ and folate

Iron

Food iron. A normal mixed diet supplies about 14 mg of iron each day of which only 1–2 mg (5–10 per cent) are absorbed. The iron is present either as *inorganic iron* (trivalent ferric iron, Fe^{+++} and divalent ferrous iron, Fe^{++}) or iron in *haem*, generally the haem of myoglobin in meat. In the stomach inorganic iron complexes to various substances including protein and polysaccharides and these iron complexes are called chelates. The acid in the gastric juice helps to keep some iron in a soluble form. On the whole the overall composition of the diet determines how much iron is available for absorption. Iron is poorly absorbed in the presence of some food such as eggs, but better absorbed with others such as milk and meat.

Absorption. Absorption of iron takes place in the upper 40 cm of small gut. Inorganic and haem iron are absorbed by different mechanisms. Haem enters the mucosal cells lining the gut and the iron is split from the haem in the cell. The absorption of haem iron is not affected by factors interfering with or promoting absorption of inorganic iron.

The amount of inorganic iron that is absorbed is regulated by the epithelial cells lining the intestine. Iron from the diet enters the mucosal cell and in the first instance is present in the cell sap where it may be linked to a protein. Some of the iron may be needed by the cell itself and this is incorporated into mitochondria in the cell. The remaining iron either passes through to the portal blood (and is absorbed) or is held in the cell by apoferritin. When iron is wanted by the body the ferritin content of the cell is low or absent so that all the iron entering the cell is passed on. If the body has enough iron, ferritin is produced within the cell and most of the iron coming in is trapped by the ferritin (Fig. 4.1). When the epithelial cell comes to the end of its life span (3–4 days) the cell with its entrapped iron is cast off, back into the gut lumen. This has been called the 'mucosal block'.

Entry of inorganic iron into the mucosal cell is promoted by reducing substances (ascorbic acid, cysteine), hydrochloric acid and succinic acid. It is inhibited by phytates and phosphates in food.

Control of iron absorption. Iron has been described as a 'one-way substance'. It is absorbed but there are no mechanisms for significant excretion. On the contrary there are elaborate mechanisms for conserving and retaining body iron (Ch. 3). The body has 3000–4000 mg of iron and normal absorption is about 1–2 mg. This exactly balances unavoidable iron loss associated with the normal shedding of skin and gut cells and the additional loss of iron during menstruation in women. Thus iron balance is controlled by the regulation of the amount absorbed from the gut.

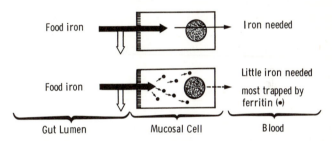

Fig. 4.1 Role of the intestinal cell in regulating iron absorption. Normally some of the iron entering the cell is held by ferritin and not allowed to pass to portal blood. In iron lack there is very little ferritin in the cell so that most of the iron entering the cell is able to pass through. Iron trapped in the cell is passed back to the gut when the cell is shed from the tip of the villus.

The mechanism whereby the intestinal cell releases or traps entering iron is the ferritin content of the cell. The amount of ferritin in turn may be determined by the amount of iron entering the cell from the 'body end'. Where there is a high marrow demand for iron it may be that less iron reaches the dividing gut epithelial cell from plasma which then has a lower ferritin content. When there is a lower marrow demand more plasma iron reaches the dividing gut cell, and more ferritin is produced indicating a smaller requirement for iron. Iron absorption is increased not only in response to iron lack but also in response to increased marrow activity.

Plasma iron transport. Four mg of iron are present in plasma carried on a specific protein, a β-globulin, called transferrin. Most of the iron entering plasma comes from the break-down of red cells and much less from body stores and from the gut. Most of this iron is going to the erythroid cells in the marrow. There is no free iron in the body.

There are at least 18 types of transferrin which are transmitted genetically and which differ in their electrophoretic mobility.

Transferrin is synthesized in the liver, each molecule of transferrin being capable of carrying two atoms of iron. It may be that the two iron receptors on transferrin have different functions, the one donating iron to marrow and placenta, and the other to iron stores as in liver (Fig. 4.2).

Normally plasma has sufficient transferrin to carry 300 μg iron per 100 ml (range 260 to 400 μg/100 ml) (54– range 47–72 μmol/l). This value is also called total iron-binding capacity. One third of the transferrin carries iron—that is, the plasma iron level is 100 μg/100 ml (18 μmol/l) so that transferrin is normally one third saturated (range 60 to 160 μg/100 ml or 11–29 μmol/l). Transferrin is present not only in plasma but in all other body fluids. It is measured by iron uptake or by an immuno-assay.

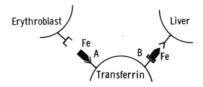

Fig. 4.2 Transferrin binds two iron atoms. Once receptor (A) may donate iron to marrow and the other (B) to iron stores.

Reticulocytes take up iron from transferrin and incorporate this iron into haemoglobin. Transferrin attaches to the reticulocyte surface, there is a rapid transfer of iron from transferrin to the cell and the transferrin then leaves the cell surface. It is presumed that a similar sequence occurs in erythroblasts in the marrow.

Plasma ferritin may also be a significant transport vehicle for iron and in particular in transporting iron derived from the breakdown of haemoglobin.

In marrow, erythroblasts may be observed encircling iron-storage reticulum cells. It has been suggested probably incorrectly that the erythroblasts are obtaining ferritin molecules (see later) from the reticulum cell by direct transfer. This process has been given the strange name of ropheocytosis. It is more probable that the transfer of iron is in the opposite direction and that erythroblasts are disposing of surplus iron by this means.

Storage iron, ferritin and haemosiderin. In a healthy man about a quarter of the iron in the body may be storage iron. In women this is usually far smaller in amount and many healthy women have little demonstrable iron stores. Iron stores can be demonstrated by staining a tissue such as marrow by Perls prussian blue method which gives a blue-green colour with iron aggregates. This is seen in marrow fragments under low power where the iron is held in tissue macrophages. In addition iron granules may be seen in the cytoplasm of erythroblasts, and erythroblasts stained in this way are termed sideroblasts. These are normal cells.

The protein storing iron is made up of 24 units to form a shell with iron atoms on the inside. The iron-free protein is called apoferritin, that containing iron is ferritin. Each ferritin molecule can hold up to 4000 iron atoms stored as ferric iron. Iron readily goes in and out of the shell, the most recent iron being the first to leave.

The development of a radioimmune assay for ferritin has expanded our knowledge about this compound considerably. It is a normal component of serum and all body cells. In healthy adults the concentration of ferritin in serum is related to the available storage iron in the body and ranges from 12 to 250 μg per litre. The normal distribution is skewed so that there is a long tail of higher values. It is below 12 μg per litre in iron deficiency and raised in iron overload. Serum ferritin at least is closely related to macrophage (reticuloendothelial) ferritin and its synthesis is stimulated by the appearance of iron in the cell. Ferritins are composed of different isoproteins termed isoferritins and different types may be present in the same organ. They are distinguished by differing electrophoretic mobilities and by isoelectric focussing.

Haemosiderin is thought to be a degradation product of ferritin. Iron stores are present throughout the body, the liver and marrow being major storage sites. Storage iron is taken up by transferrin for transfer to developing erythroblasts when required.

Ferrokinetics

^{59}Fe is an isotope with a half life of 45 days which emits high energy gamma rays so that it is possible to trace its distribution in the body by holding a counter over appropriate positions. Useful information about how iron is used may be obtained by adding a tracer dose of ^{59}Fe to the subject's plasma so that it binds to transferrin, and returning the plasma to the subject's circulation.

Plasma iron clearance. The ^{59}Fe will normally leave transferrin to be taken up by tissues such as marrow, half the dose being gone in about 90 minutes.

Surface counting. The disappearance of plasma ^{59}Fe is accompanied by a rising level of ^{59}Fe iron in the marrow in the three hours following administration of the dose. This is assessed by placing the external counter over the sacrum (which represents marrow) as compared with blood (counter over the heart). As the iron is utilized for haemoglobin synthesis over the next 10 days the sacral radioactivity falls and that over the heart rises (Fig. 4.3).

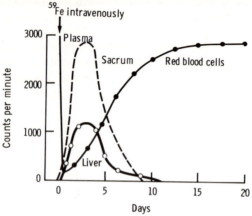

Fig. 4.3 Injected ^{59}Fe disappears from plasma in a few hours to marrow ($\equiv$sacrum) and thereafter reappears in haemoglobin in newly formed red cells over the next 10 days. These counts are obtained by holding a counter over the heart ($\equiv$ *blood*), liver and sacrum. Blood samples are collected after the injection for plasma counts.

Utilization of iron. The ^{59}Fe increasingly appears in the red cells to reach a plateau after 10 days. At this point between 70–90 per cent of the ^{59}Fe has been used for haemoglobin synthesis.

Plasma iron turnover. The amount of iron passing through plasma over 24 hours can be calculated from knowledge of the ^{59}Fe clearance, serum iron level and plasma volume. The normal value is 38 mg/24 hours.

Iron absorption. A further variant of these tests is to give the ^{59}Fe orally. Iron absorption can then be assessed by the manner in which the oral iron appears in red cells as well as by noting how much iron is retained within the body using a whole body counter. Unabsorbed iron can be assessed by the radioactivity in the faeces, but as relatively little iron is normally absorbed this is an unreliable method.

Function of iron. Most of the iron goes to the synthesis of haemoglobin. Iron is also required for myoglobin of muscle and for enzymes like xanthine oxidase and succinic dehydrogenase and other enzymes like aconitase.

Iron requirements are between 1–2 mg per day, that is, enough to meet daily losses. Growing children and menstruating women require more than adult males. In the latter two thirds of normal pregnancy daily iron requirements increase to 4–6 mg daily.

Vitamin B$_{12}$

Structure. Vitamin B$_{12}$ or cobalamin has a structure that is similar to the haem moiety of haemoglobin (Fig. 4.4). It too consists of four pyrrole groups but these four are linked to a cobalt atom. This structure is called the corrin nucleus.

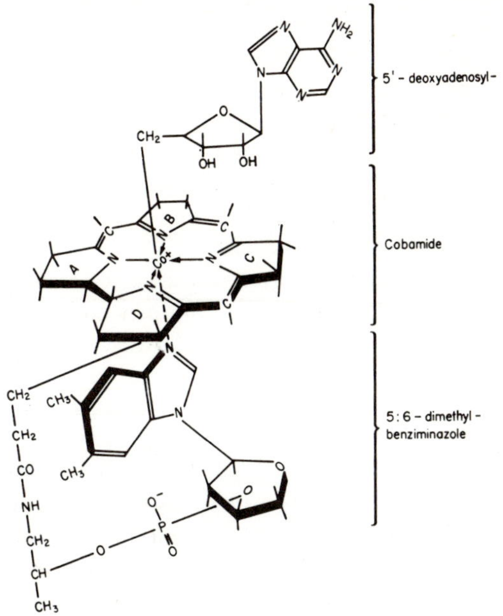

Fig. 4.4 Vitamin B$_{12}$. The altered pyrrole ring (A, B, C and D) are linked to cobalt. An unusual nucleotide, benzimidazole is present and in the coenzyme form, adenosine.

Dietary sources. The primary source of cobalamins is bacterial synthesis. Higher animals must obtain the preformed vitamin. Ruminants, that is grass eating animals having a foregut, meet their vitamin B$_{12}$ needs from synthesis of cobalamins by bacteria normally resident in the foregut. Man obtains vitamin B$_{12}$ from foodstuffs of animal origin including milk, eggs, meat etc. Water may have trace amounts of vitamin B$_{12}$ and foods such as yogurt have additional vitamin B$_{12}$ from the bacterial activity in the milk. Vitamin B$_{12}$ is not required by the plant kingdom and vegetables and fruits are totally devoid of vitamin B$_{12}$.

A normal mixed diet provides an average of 5 μg of vitamin B$_{12}$ daily. A vegetarian diet will contain very little—generally well below 1 μg per day, and that amount is probably due to bacterial contamination of food.

Requirements and body stores. Each day some 2–4 μg of vitamin B_{12} are lost or degraded in the body. The replacement of this daily loss constitutes man's normal requirements. The body stores in subjects taking a mixed diet, are about 3000 μg (3 mg). Strict vegetarians have very low vitamin B_{12} stores. Most of the vitamin B_{12} is in the liver, which in man contains 1 μg of vitamin B_{12} per gram.

Intrinsic factor. This is a glycoprotein (MW 55000) necessary for the absorption of vitamin B_{12}. Each molecule of intrinsic factor binds to one molecule of vitamin B_{12}.

The body of the stomach has a variety of specialized secreting cells. On the surface are mucus-secreting cells. Beneath the surface lie columns of cells which are of two types—the chief cell produces a protein-splitting enzyme, pepsinogen, and the parietal cell produces intrinsic factor and hydrochloric acid.

Intrinsic factor can be assayed by a radio-immunoassay. The amount secreted normally is about a 100 times more than is required for vitamin B_{12} absorption and is a further example of normal physiological reserve. The secretion of intrinsic factor and HCl (both from parietal cells) is stimulated by the hormone gastrin, by synthetic gastrin analogues such as pentagastrin, by histamine and insulin.

Virtually all the vitamin B_{12} in food is available for absorption. The attachment of vitamin B_{12} to intrinsic factor is very rapid and in solution is largely complete in seconds. It takes place over a wide range of pH and in the stomach this can range from near neutrality to extreme acidity (pH 1).

Unlike vitamin B_{12} intrinsic factor is labile, being destroyed by proteolytic digestion even in the stomach and by heat. Once the vitamin B_{12}-intrinsic factor complex has formed however, the situation changes. The complex is relatively resistant to proteolytic enzymes. This is important because the complex has to traverse the whole length of the gut unaltered to reach the site of vitamin B_{12} absorption in the distal small gut (ileum).

Vitamin B_{12} absorption. The normal small gut in man is over 7 metres (21 feet) in length and vitamin B_{12} is absorbed over the last 2–3 meters (6–8 feet). In this region of distal gut there are specific receptors which take up the vitamin B_{12}-intrinsic factor complex. The number of such receptors limits the amount of vitamin B_{12} that is absorbed at any one time—in practice this means that about 2 μg is the maximum amount of vitamin B_{12} that can be taken up from a single meal. With three meals per day a maximum of 6 μg vitamin B_{12} can be absorbed daily.

There is a slow separation of vitamin B_{12} from intrinsic factor in or on the epithelial cells lining the ileal villi. Vitamin B$_{12}$ alone reaches the blood in the portal veins draining the gut after a delay of 3–4 hours with maximum blood levels being reached 8–12 hours after the oral dose has been given. The carrier protein transcobalamin II (TCII) is synthesized in the ileal enterocytes and TCII-B$_{12}$ passes to the portal blood.

The cobalt in vitamin B$_{12}$ can be replaced by radioactive isotopes of Co. This is done by growing the bacterium from which vitamin B$_{12}$ is derived, in the presence of either ^{57}Co or ^{58}Co as the sole source of cobalt. Such labelled vitamin B$_{12}$ can be used to measure the intestinal absorption of vitamin B$_{12}$ in man by a number of methods.

a. After a dose of ^{57}Co- or ^{58}Co-B$_{12}$ by mouth, all the faeces are collected for six days. Unabsorbed vitamin B$_{12}$ is measured by counting radioactivity in faeces. More than half of a 1·0 μg dose is normally absorbed less than half remaining in the faeces.

b. After an oral dose of labelled vitamin B$_{12}$ the amount retained in the body can be measured by whole body counting. Again more than half of a 1·0 μg dose is normally retained.

c. The radioactivity appearing in the plasma 8 to 12 hours after an oral dose of labelled vitamin B$_{12}$ may be measured.

d. The commonest method used to assess vitamin B$_{12}$ absorption is to measure excretion of labelled vitamin B$_{12}$ in the urine (Urinary excretion or Schilling test). An injection of 1000 μg of cyanocobalamin is given with the oral labelled dose. Some of the injected vitamin B$_{12}$ saturates the transcobalamins (see later) and the rest is excreted into the urine. Almost exactly one third of labelled vitamin B$_{12}$ *absorbed from the gut* reaches the liver, recirculates and is excreted into the urine. The result is expressed as a percentage of the oral dose in the urine in 24 hours. Normally it is greater than 10 per cent with a 1·0 μg oral dose.

Transport in plasma. Vitamin B$_{12}$ in plasma is attached to two proteins located electrophoretically in the α and β globulin region. These are called transcobalamins. Most of the native vitamin B$_{12}$ in plasma is present on the larger MW (120 000) transcobalamin I, but some is also present on transcobalamin II (MW 35 000). The vitamin B$_{12}$ on transcobalamin II is rapidly given up to tissues such as the liver, but that on transcobalamin I is retained for a much longer period of time.

The transcobalamins turn over at a rapid rate, their rapid secretion into plasma ensuring that free B$_{12}$ cannot exist under normal circumstances.

A vitamin B_{12}-binding protein immunologically identical to transcobalamin I (R binder) is present in cells, all body fluids and secretions. Its physiological function is unknown. Transcobalamin II is synthesized in the liver as well as gut cells and macrophages. R-binder arises principally from white blood cells but probably also to a lesser extent from other tissues.

The amount of vitamin B_{12} present in plasma or serum can be measured either by microbiological assay or by saturation analysis techniques. The normal range depends on the method of analysis. It is usually between 160 to 1000 pg/ml.

Function of vitamin B_{12}. The vitamin is essential in man for normal blood production and for normal function of nerve tissue. Its precise role in biochemical terms is not certain.

a. It is needed for normal folic-acid coenzyme activity in cells. When vitamin B_{12} is lacking the folic-acid coenzyme level is abnormally low. The precise explanation for low folate coenzyme activity is not certain.

b. Vitamin B_{12} is needed to convert homocysteine to methionine (Fig. 4.5). This involves the addition of a CH_3 (methyl) group. Folic acid participates in this reaction so that the CH_3 (from methylfolate) is passed on to vitamin B_{12} (as methyl-B_{12}) and then transferred to homocysteine.

c. Vitamin B_{12} is needed to convert methylmalonic acid to succinic acid. This involves straightening out a carbon chain (Fig. 4.6). Methylmalonic acid arises from the three-carbon fatty acid, propionic acid and from aminoacids leucine, isoleucine and valine.

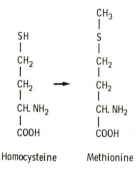

Fig. 4.5 The conversion of homocysteine to methionine requires both vitamin B_{12} and folate.

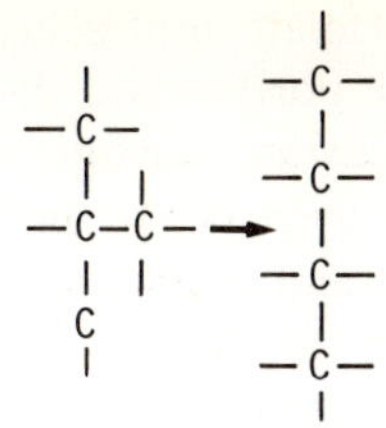

Methylmalonic   Succinic
acid   acid

Fig. 4.6 The conversion of methylmalonic acid to succinic acid involves the straightening out of a carbon chain. Vitamin B$_{12}$ carries out a similar function in a number of pathways. Only the one involving methylmalonic acid occurs in mammals.

Folate

Structure. The basic structure of this family of compounds is shown in Fig. 4.7. This is pteroylglutamic acid. Three types of change take place to this basic structure.

a. Most forms of folate have not one but usually five or six glutamic acid groups forming a peptide chain. These are termed pteroyl*poly*-glutamates.

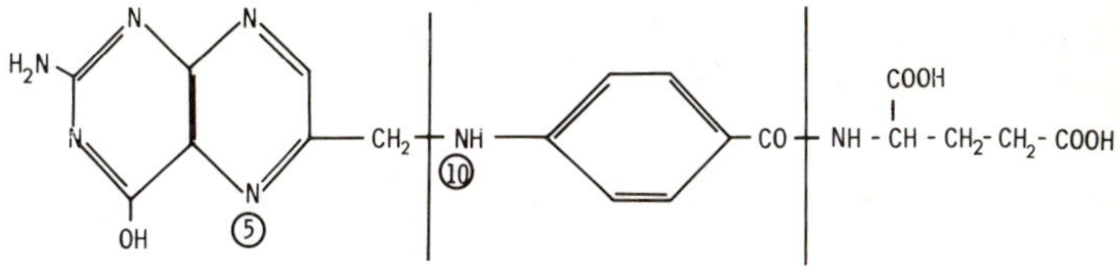

pteridine   para-amino-benzoic acid   glutamic acid

Fig. 4.7 Pteroylglutamic acid.

b. All physiological forms are reduced, having an extra two or four hydrogen atoms in the pteridine ring. These forms are termed dihydro- or tetrahydro-folates.

c. An additional carbon unit is present in the 5 or 10 position or held as a bridge between the 5 and 10 positions. The commoner forms are a methyl group (CH_3) in position 5 or a formyl (CHO) in position 10.

Dietary sources. Folates are widely distributed in foodstuffs of both plant and animal origin. Some three quarters of the folate in food are polyglutamate forms and all are reduced. A normal mixed diet supplies between 200 to 400 μg folate daily.

Unlike vitamin B$_{12}$, natural folates are easily destroyed the molecule being split into the pteridine portion and the para-aminobenzoate. This is brought about by oxidation and agents include atmospheric oxygen, heat and ultraviolet light. Thus the folate content of food steadily declines with storage and drops abruptly with cooking.

Requirement is between 100–200 μg daily and in pregnancy between 200–300 μg daily. The total amount of folate in the body of a normal adult is between 10–20 mg.

Absorption. Dietary folates are absorbed by an active process generally from the upper half of the small gut. During the passage of folate through the intestinal cell the molecule is altered so that normally only 5-methyltetrahydrofolate appears in the blood (Fig. 4.8).

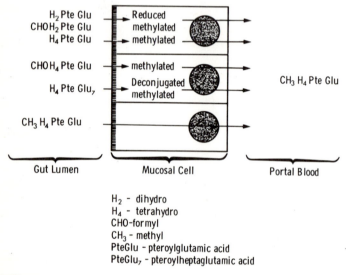

H$_2$ Pte Glu
CHOH$_2$ Pte Glu
H$_4$ Pte Glu

CHOH$_4$ Pte Glu
H$_4$ Pte Glu$_7$

CH$_3$ H$_4$ Pte Glu

Reduced
methylated
methylated

methylated
Deconjugated
methylated

CH$_3$ H$_4$ Pte Glu

Gut Lumen   Mucosal Cell   Portal Blood

H$_2$ – dihydro
H$_4$ – tetrahydro
CHO-formyl
CH$_3$ – methyl
PteGlu – pteroylglutamic acid
PteGlu$_7$ – pteroylheptaglutamic acid

4.8 The absorption of folate. All natural folates are reduced. In the intestinal cell it is further reduced (if necessary) to tetrahydrofolate, a single carbon is added probably as formate, and this is reduced to methyl and finally 5-methyltetrahydropteroylglutamic acid enters portal blood. Polyglutamate forms of folate, in addition, have glutamic acid residues in excess of one, removed.

In the case of the polyglutamate forms, the molecule is taken into the intestinal epithelial cell and the glutamic acid chain removed to leave a monoglutamate. The enzyme responsible for this is *folate conjugase*. This enzyme is in the lysosomes of the cell and its pH optimum is 4·5. Any partially reduced forms of folate that enter the cell are reduced to tetrahydrofolates and the enzyme responsible is called *dihydrofolate reductase.* Finally, an extra carbon is added, probably as a formyl group and then the carbon further reduced to methyl.

Normally over 90 per cent of monoglutamates are absorbed and a lesser (but as yet uncertain) proportion of polyglutamate forms.

The absorption of folate can be tested by giving an oral dose and measuring the rise in the serum folic acid level over the next two hours. Before doing such a test it is necessary to give folic acid to the subject for a few days to obtain standard clearance of absorbed folate from blood to tissues. An alternative method is to give tritium-labelled folic acid by mouth and, at the same time 15 mg of ordinary folic acid by injection. The urine is then collected for 24 hours and tritium in the urine counted.

Serum and red cell folate. Methyltetrahydrofolate is present in normal serum (or plasma) and methyltetrahydropenta- and hexa-glutamates in red cells. These may be measured by microbiological assay. Following haemolysis of whole blood, the folate polyglutamates in the red cells react with a conjugase enzyme normally present in plasma to release a monoglutamate. This is necessary because the microbiological assay organisms can only use monoglutamates and short chain polyglutamates.

Normal serum folate is 3–15 ng/ml and red cell folate 150–500 ng/ml packed red cells.

Function of folate. Folate functions as a co-enzyme (i.e. works together with a protein enzyme) in the transfer of single carbon units in a number of important pathways. The carbon units transferred are $-CH_3$ (methyl), $-CH_2$ (methylene), $-CH=$(methenyl) or $-CHO$ (formyl). The source of the carbon is generally the 3 carbon aminoacid, serine, which gets changed to the 2 carbon aminoacid, glycine. The reactions are:

a. Synthesis of thymidine by adding an extra carbon to de-oxyuridine.
b. Synthesis of purine. Two of the carbons in the purine nucleus arrive via folate.

   Thymidine and purines are required for the deoxyribosenucleic acid (DNA) of cell nuclei and purines are required for the ribosenucleic acid (RNA). These compounds are synthesized in dividing and growing cells; not only the blood cells but all tissues that renew themselves including skin, the lining of the mouth, the gut, kidney tubules, bladder surfaces etc.
c. Formation of methionine from homocysteine.
d. Minor pathways involve the conversion of histidine to glutamic acid. An intermediate is formiminoglutamic acid (Figlu). The

formimino group is –CH=NH and this is normally passed on to tetrahydrofolic acid (Fig. 4.9).

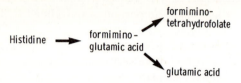

Fig. 4.9 Histidine is converted to formiminoglutamic acid. The forminino (–CH=NH) group is transferred to tetrahydrofolic acid leaving glutamic acid.

Other requirements for normal erythropoiesis

Lack of iron, vitamin B_{12} and folate often lead to a failure of normal blood production. The composition of red cells is as complex as other body tissues and many other materials are required in their production. Lack of these other components only rarely occurs in clinical practice and thus leads to anaemia only very rarely. Aminoacids, lipids and carbohydrates are required. Vitamins functioning as co-enzymes include riboflavin, pantothenic acid, niacin, pyridoxine, thiamine, biotin, tocopherol (Vitamin E) and ascorbic acid (Vitamin C).

Minerals in trace amount include zinc and copper. Normal endocrine function is necessary including thyroid and adrenal hormones.

References

Chanarin I 1979 The Megaloblastic Anaemias, 2nd edn, Blackwell, Oxford
Jacobs A and Worwood M 1975 New England Journal of Medicine: 951–956

5

Biochemical systems in blood cells

Red blood cells

The mature red cell does not have a nucleus and as a result is not able to synthesize new proteins including enzymes. The reticulocyte still has considerable synthetic activity, e.g. it can make new globin chains and incorporate iron into haemoglobin. The red cell possesses a number of enzyme systems and when these 'wear out' the cell is removed. The enzyme systems are needed so that the red cell can maintain its normal shape and flexibility, maintain the iron in haem in the ferrous (Fe^{++}) state and maintain its normal internal biochemical and electrolyte composition.

Biochemical systems in red cells are concerned with

a. Utilization of glucose to provide energy (ATP) –Embden–Meyerhof pathway.
b. Utilization of glucose to produce reducing agents (NADPH) –Pentose–phosphate pathway.
c. Changing the affinity of haemoglobin for oxygen –Diphosphoglycerate enzymes.
d. Maintaining reduced haemoglobin –Methaemoglobin reductase and glutathione reductase.
e. Some phases of pyrimidine and purine nucleotide synthesis and others.

The red cell membrane. Analysis of red cell ghosts show a protein skeleton in the form of a regular network of fibrils like a hair net on EM and composed largely of a protein which has been termed spectrin but with smaller amounts of a second protein called actin. This mesh is present on the inside of the membrane. On this mesh are some layers of lipid with phosphates on the inner and outer surfaces and fatty acid chains directed to the middle. Glycoproteins traverse the membrane at various sites. About half the mass of the membrane is composed of lipid and although there is no synthesis of new lipid, there is considerable exchange of membrane cholesterol, free fatty acid and phosphatides with that in plasma. In addition the red cell membrane is able to acylate some of these lipids using adenosinetriphosphate (ATP).

The membrane surface is also the site of various antigens detectable in blood-grouping serology. Other proteins are adsorbed on to the surface of the red cell from the plasma, the best example being the Lewis blood group substance. Many of the enzymes in the red cell are located in the red cell membrane.

Water, glucose, lactose and electrolytes readily pass through the red cell membrane. There is less sodium and about 20 times more potassium in the red cell than in plasma. An energy-requiring mechanism is concerned with maintaining these levels, that is, energy is required to pump out sodium and to keep potassium in the red cell.

Anaerobic glycolysis (Embden–Meyerhof). This is the pathway by which glucose is used for the release of energy. The red cell membrane has a specific carrier system to get glucose into the cell. A simplified version of the breakdown of glucose to lactose is shown in Fig. 5.1.

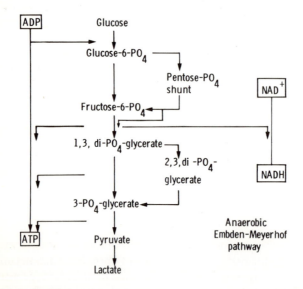

Fig. 5.1 A simplified version of the Embden-Meyerhof pathway for the anaerobic utilization of glucose.

Lactose finally diffuses out of the red cell and is utilized further elsewhere. Energy in the red cell is locked up in adenosine triphosphate (ATP). Removal of one phosphate to give adenosine diphosphate (ADP) simultaneously releases the energy needed within the red cell (called high energy phosphate bond). Each molecule of glucose degraded, finally gives rise to two molecules of ATP. Thus the function of the glycolytic pathway is the maintenance of the intracellular red cell ATP level. Ninety per cent of the glucose used in the red cells follow this pathway.

In addition to supplying ATP the anaerobic glycolytic pathway yields supplies of reduced nicotinamide adenine dinucleotide (NADH) from the oxidized form (NAD^+). This compound in conjunction with the enzyme methaemoglobin reductase, is important in the conversion of methaemoglobin (Fe^{+++}) to haemoglobin (Fe^{++}).

Aerobic glycolysis (Pentose-phosphate pathway). Normally only about 10 per cent of the glucose is metabolized along this pathway. The starting point is glucose-6-phosphate. One of the carbons of glucose-6-phosphate becomes oxidized to carbon dioxide (CO_2). This pathway (Fig. 5.2) provides all the reduced nicotinamide adenine dinucleotide phosphate (NADPH) in the red cell. NADPH is needed to keep glutathione (GSSG) in the reduced state (GSH). This pathway does *not* provide 'energy'.

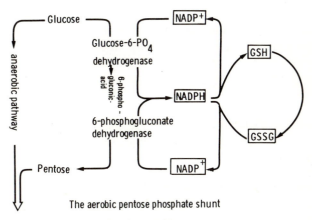

The aerobic pentose phosphate shunt

Fig. 5.2 The aerobic pentose-phosphate pathway.

The amount of glucose metabolized in this pathway is probably regulated by the amount of $NADP^+$ that has accumulated. Glutathione itself is probably synthesized in the red cell. Reduced glutathione (GSH) is concerned with the disposal of hydrogen peroxide which otherwise would oxidize haemoglobin to methaemoglobin. The enzyme which shunts glucose-6-PO_4 into the aerobic pathway is called glucose-6-phosphate dehydrogenase (G-6PD). The pentose which is formed finally re-enters the Embden-Meyerhof path as fructose and glyceraldehyde.

Reducing systems in red cells. Normally a small amount of haemoglobin is constantly being oxidized with the formation of methaemoglobin. When this happens, ferrous iron (Fe^{++}) is changed to ferric iron (Fe^{+++}). Many drugs used therapeutically hasten this change. The red cell is equipped with reducing systems that convert methaemoglobin back to the ferrous state and normally oxidation and reduction of haemoglobin are in balance. Enzymatic reduction of methaemoglobin is carried out by methaemoglobin reductase (also called NADH-diaphorase or NADH-dehydrogenase). Non-enzymatic reduction of methaemoglobin is less important but may occur via the agency of reduced glutathione (GSH) and even ascorbic acid.

Glutathione which is present in relatively high concentration in red cells and with the enzyme glutathione peroxidase, converts hydrogen peroxide (H_2O_2) to water. Hydrogen peroxide forms spontaneously in red cells and is produced in increased amount after drug medication. A second enzyme, catalase, is also capable of breakdown of H_2O_2 but nevertheless red cells totally lacking catalase, survive normally and hence catalase is probably not important.

Role of 2,3-diphosphoglycerate (2,3-DPG). The oxygen affinity of haemoglobin is inversely proportional to the concentration of this compound in the red cell (Ch. 3). DPG binds to the β-globin chain of haemoglobin. It is produced during the course of glucose breakdown by the action of the enzyme, disphosphoglyceromutase on 1,3 diphosphoglycerate.

Nucleic acid synthesis. Although incapable of the overall synthesis of purines and pyrimidines red cells retain several enzymes concerned with producing these compounds. Adenosine may be used by red cells to produce a high-energy phosphate bond and addition of this compound to blood has been used to preserve blood for transfusion.

Other enzymes. Red cells contain carbonic anhydrase which is concerned with CO_2 transport in and out of the cell, and acetylcholinesterase the role of which is uncertain.

Granulocytes

Mature granulocytes are able to synthesize protein as judged by the incorporation of labelled aminoacids. Purines and pyrimidines can be synthesized and preformed compounds re-utilized. Both proteins and nucleic acids can be catabolized by mature granulocytes.

Leucocyte alkaline phosphatase (LAP) is a zinc-containing enzyme catalyzing the hydrolysis of a wide range of phosphoester substrates.

LAP is first detectable in neutrophil myelocytes and its activity increases with cell maturity. Its function *in vivo* is not known. Its activity increases in infections possibly due to increased release of corticosteroids and decreases in leukaemic states as well as in glandular fever, idiopathic thrombocytopenia and paroxysmal nocturnal haemoglobinuria.

Energy in granulocytes is derived mainly from oxidation of glucose to lactate both aerobic and anaerobic pathways being available. Glucose is also actively stored by conversion into glycogen. Granulocytes have relatively few mitochondria and hence the activity of the citric acid cycle is relatively low and less than 5 per cent of glucose is oxidized to CO_2 via this cycle. The cells are capable of active lipid synthesis.

The levels of several vitamins have been measured in granulocytes particularly ascorbic acid, folic acid, pyridoxal phosphate, thiamine, riboflavin and B_{12} and B_{12}-binding proteins are present.

The specific granules of neutrophils contain lysozyme, collagenase and alkaline phosphatase and the azurophil primary granules acid hydrolases and peroxidase.

The large granules of eosinophil granulocytes contains a mucopolysaccharide, and lysosomal (hydrolytic) enzymes, peroxidase, phospholipase and an arylsulphatase. The eosinophilic staining is due to a high content of cationic protein.

Neutrophils engaged in phagocytosis produce superoxide, that is reactive O and hydrogen peroxide probably in the region of the cell surface. These substances are toxic to bacteria. The superoxide itself is converted to hydrogen peroxide. A lactoferrin which chelates iron may, by so doing, remove a bacterial growth factor.

Platelets

The *platelet membrane* has the usual constitutents of cell membranes, protein (57 per cent) and lipid (33 per cent) being the principal components, with carbohydrates (8 per cent) making up most of the remaining dry weight. Three quarters of the lipids are phospholipids, the named constituents including arachidonic acid and a factor associated with platelet factor 3 activity. Arachidonic acid, after release by phospholipase, is converted into oxygenated products including prostaglandins.

Three glycoproteins (I, II and III) have been identified in the membrane and these are abnormal in thrombasthenic states. The platelet membrane is also the site of a large number of enzymes including phosphodiesterase, acid phosphatase, ATPase, 5-nucleotidase and adenylate cyclase.

The *platelet cytoplasm* contains fibrinogen located in granules, probably synthetized by the megakaryocytes, and this constitutes about 13 per cent of platelet protein. The platelet contractile protein, an actinomyosine-like protein called thrombasthenin, is present in both membrane and cytoplasm.

Among enzymes present in the granules are acid hydrolases, peptidases, neuraminidase, cathepsin, catalase and acetylcholin-esterase. The granules also contain low molecular weight peptides such as platelet factor 4 (heparin-neutralizing activity) and β-thromboglobulin.

Glycogen is the major carbohydrate in the cytoplasm and is probably made in the platelet via glycogen synthetase. The hexo-semonophosphate shunt is present leading to the production of NADPH necessary for the biosynthesis of fatty acids and conversion of pyruvate and lactate to hexose.

Adenosine, guanosine, uridine and cytidine are present, as well as large amounts of ADP and ATP. ADP and ATP are present as a metabolic pool and a storage pool. The storage pool is situated in the dense granules and is released during secretion. The ATP in the metabolic pool turns over continuously to provide energy for various functions including membrane transport and synthetic reactions.

Platelets also possess cyclic AMP and their relation to prostaglandins and the vessel wall is discussed in Chapter 6.

References

Beutler E 1977 In: Williams J W, Buetler E, Erslev A J, Rundles R W (eds) Haematology 2nd edn. McGraw-Hill, New York, p. 117–190

Crawford N, Taylor D G 1977 Biochemical aspects of platelet behaviour. British Medical Bulletin 33: 199–206

Holmsen H, Salganicoff L, Fukami M H 1977 Platelet behaviour and Biochemistry. In: Ogston D, Bennett B (eds) Haemostasis; biochemistry, physiology and pathology. John Wiley and Sons, London, p 239–319

6

Haemostasis

Haemostasis is the process of arresting bleeding from an injured blood vessel. It is due in the first instance to constriction of the vessel wall and is followed by closing the site of blood leakage by a haemostatic plug which consists of platelets and fibrin in which red cells and granulocytes are trapped. Blood flow, plasma inhibitors and fibrinolysis prevent uncontrolled growth of the haemostatic plug; fibrinolysis finally removes the fibrin strands when tissue repair is complete. Haemostasis is thus achieved through an interaction of the vessel wall, platelets and coagulation. In small blood vessels platelets play the crucial role, whereas in large vessels coagulation of blood is the most important factor. Haemostasis is shown schematically in figure 6.1.

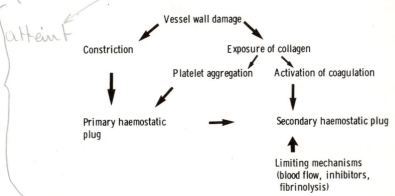

Fig. 6.1 An outline of normal haemostasis.

Blood vessels

A typical blood vessel has an inner layer, the intima, a middle layer, the media and an outer layer, the adventitia (Fig. 6.2).

The *intima*, the inner layer of the vessel, consists of flat endothelial cells. These cells synthesize and release factor VIII antigen (the protein part of factor VIII molecule), PGI_2 (a prostaglandin that inhibits platelet aggregation), antithrombin III (an inhibitor of plasma serine proteases) and plasminogen activator, an enzyme that initiates fibrinolysis. Between media and intima is the subendothelium which consists of a basement membrane, microfibrils of elastin and amorphous elastin. Platelets will adhere to the first two of these structures.

The next layer, the *media*, has collagen fibres, smooth muscle cells and fibroblasts. Collagen is a protein that initiates rapid platelet adhesion and secretion; it also activates factor XII which in turn starts the coagulation sequence and fibrinolysis. The outer layer of the vessel is the *adventitia* which consists of connective tissue carrying nerves and nutrient blood vessels.

Schematic representation of blood vessel

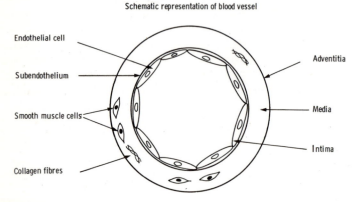

Fig. 6.2 Cross section of a blood vessel showing the inner layer (intima), middle layer (media) and outer layer (adventitia).

Constriction of larger blood vessels in response to injury is due to contraction of smooth muscle cells. Closure of smaller blood vessels may involve endothelial adhesion or a precapillary sphincter.

Platelets

Platelets participate in the arrest of bleeding by plugging the disrupted vessel wall and by providing components essential for coagulation. These two functions are closely interrelated.

Platelets have an average volume of about seven fl. On light microscopy their structure appears extremely simple with transparent cytoplasm and a central darkly stained granular area (hyalomere). On electron microscopy the structure is more complex (Fig. 6.3).

The *peripheral zone* is the site of platelet adhesion and aggregation. The surface contains receptors for thrombin, collagen, ADP, adrenaline and serotonin. Many plasma proteins and coagulation factors V, XI and fibrinogen are tightly bound to the surface. Within the platelet is the *sol-gel zone* which contains microtubules and microfilaments both composed of thrombasthenin. The microtubules are arranged along the greatest circumference of the platelet. The *organelles* include mitochondria, dense bodies, larger granules, glycogen and the Golgi apparatus. Dense bodies and granules are released into plasma during the release reaction through the open canalicular system.

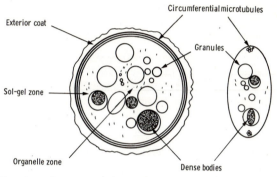

Fig. 6.3 The schematic structure of a platelet as seen on electron microscopy.

The different phases of platelet function are termed *adhesion, aggregation, contraction,* and *secretion* (release). **Adhesion** is the interaction of platelets with the damaged vessel wall. The interaction of platelets with each other is called aggregation and can be initiated by thrombin, collagen, ADP, free fatty acids, adrenaline, serotonin, and immune complexes, as well as many other substances. Often these phases of platelet reaction occur synchronously but they are more easily understood if each is dealt with separately. Adhesion to collagen is important for the formation of the haemostatic plug *in vivo* and induces an immediate platelet secretion related to the structural arrangement of the collagen microfibrils. Platelets also adhere to subendothelial microfibrils and this requires plasma factor VIII von Willebrand factor. There is an additional interaction between the vessel wall and platelets: prostaglandins from arachidonic acid generate an unstable substance, thromboxane A_2, which induces aggregation. On the other hand, prostaglandins are also utilized by the endothelial cells to produce PGI_2. PGI_2 inhibits further platelet aggregation. The generation of two substances with opposing biological effects from the same substrate is probably a safeguard against intravascular thrombosis.

The mechanism that enables platelets to aggregate is unclear, but it may involve coagulation on the surface of the platelet with generation of traces of thrombin, or inhibition of membrane adenyl-cyclase, an enzyme that forms cyclic AMP from ATP, or mobilization of calcium into the sol-gel zone. Thereafter ADP, released from the platelet, red cells or vessel wall, provides the impetus for further events. Even in very small concentrations ADP causes membrane changes. The platelets lose their discoid shape, and start to adhere to other platelets which results in the formation of large aggregates. With the change of shape the organelles move to the centre of the platelet. This is contraction (Fig. 6.4). *Contraction* is an energy-dependent process and is potentially reversible in which case release does not occur. The process of *release* or *secretion* is, however, irreversible. The point of no return is reached when the open canalicular system fuses with dense bodies and granules. These granules are discharged amongst the aggregated platelets and into the surrounding plasma. The two types of granules participate in two different types of secretion. Dense granules only (secretion I) are released if aggregation is induced by serotonin, adrenaline or ADP. The substances contained in dense granules are ADP, ATP, serotonin, pyrophosphate and calcium. Secretion II involves both dense granules and α granules and is induced by thrombin and collagen. α granules contain lysozymes, PF_4, β-thromboglobulin, catalase and many other factors. Serotonin is a vasoconstrictor. Platelet factor 4 neutralizes trace amounts of endogenous heparin and may thus accelerate coagulation in the vicinity of the platelet plug.

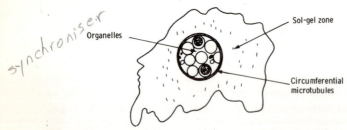

Fig. 6.4 The scheme of changes in internal platelet structure following ADP aggregation (contracted platelet) as seen on electron microscopy.

Coagulation

The coagulation sequence is the chain of reactions which lead to the formation of a fibrin clot. Coagulation factors, platelets, phospholipid and ionized calcium are necessary for blood to clot. The nomenclature of clotting factors is given in Table 1.

Coagulation occurs via two pathways each of which lead to the formation of fibrin clot.

Table 6.1   Nomenclature of clotting factors

Factor	
I	fibrinogen
II	prothrombin
III*	tissue factor
IV*	calcium
V	proaccelerin, labile factor
VII	proconvertin, stable factor
VIII	antihaemophilic factor
IX	Christmas factor, plasma thromboplastin component
X	Stuart-Prower factor
XI	plasma thromboplastin antecedent
XII	Hageman factor
XIII	fibrin-stabilizing factor

*Rarely if ever used.

The intrinsic pathway

Here (Fig. 6.5) injury to the intima exposes collagen and other subintimal components that activate Factor XII. Activated factor XII activates factor XI which in turn activates factor IX. Together with platelets, factor VIII and calcium, factor IX activates factor X. This phase of coagulation lasts 5–10 minutes and defects in this phase give rise to a long whole blood clotting time and a long kaolin-cephalin time. Some characteristics of coagulation factors participating in the intrinsic pathway are given in Table 6.2.

Factor VIII consists of at least three entities (1) factor VIII clot-promoting activity, (Factor VIIIC) lacking in haemophilia, (2) factor VIII-related antigen, a protein detectable by precipitating antisera to Factor VIII (Factor VIII RAg). Factor VIII RAg is absent in many patients with von Willebrand's syndrome but is present in haemophilia. (3) Plasma activity necessary for ristocetin-induced platelet agglutination: factor VIII von Willebrand factor, or factor VIIIVWF. Factor

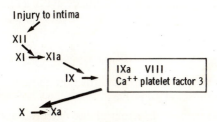

Fig. 6.5 The intrinsic pathway of blood coagulation.

Table 6.2   Coagulation factors of the intrinsic pathway

Factor	MW	Plasma concentration, μg/ml	Plasma half life	Site of synthesis	Adsorbed by
XII	90000	40	2–3 d	?liver	celite, kaolin
XI	60000	7	2–3 d	liver	celite, kaolin
IX	55000	3–4	18–36 h	liver	$BaSO_4$, $Al(OH)_3$
				vit. K. dependent	
VIII	?2000000	?	12–15 h	?	—

VIIIVWF is also responsible for controlling the bleeding time and platelet adhesion to subendothelial microfibrils and is defective in von Willebrand's disease. It is uncertain whether all three properties are carried on one molecule or whether a complicated interaction between different plasma constituents is involved.

The extrinsic pathway

In the extrinsic pathway alterations of endothelial cell membrane expose a tissue factor which activates or complexes with factor VII to activate factor X (Fig. 6.6). This sequence is very rapid and its defects result in a prolonged one stage prothrombin time.

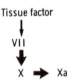

Fig. 6.6 The extrinsic pathway of blood coagulation.

The generation of thrombin

Once activated by either pathway, factor X in association with platelets and factor V, converts prothrombin into thrombin. Thrombin is a proteolytic enzyme, with amino acid serine as its active centre, that cleaves two pairs of arginine-glycine bonds in fibrinogen and converts it into fibrin monomer. This part of the coagulation sequence lasts 10–20 seconds. The defects are reflected in a prolonged one stage prothrombin time and prolonged kaolin-cephalin time (Fig. 6.7). Thrombin also activates factor XIII, transforms factor VIIIC and V into forms more active in the coagulation sequence, and induces platelet aggregation and secretion.

Some characteristics of factors of the extrinsic and the common pathway are shown in Table 6.3

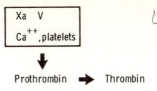

Fig. 6.7 Later stages in the coagulation sequence.

Formation of fibrin

The fibrinogen molecule is a dimer, each monomer being composed of three chains named Aα, Bβ and γ, linked by disulphide bridges (Fig. 6.8).

Thrombin cleaves fibrinopeptides A and B from fibrinogen and the remaining 'part of the molecule is called fibrin monomer. Fibrin monomers link together into fibrin polymers, which are easily lysed by fibrinolysins *in vivo* and are soluble in urea and monochloracetic acid *in vitro*. Factor XIII, activated in two steps, by thrombin and calcium, promotes the formation of crosslinks between adjacent fibrin monomers by linking ϵ-lysine and γ-glutamyl residues. This results in the formation of a stable fibrin (Fig. 6.9). Unlike the rapid action of thrombin on fibrinogen, the formation of stable fibrin is slow and complete cross-linking takes several hours. Defects in the thrombin-fibrinogen interaction are reflected in all the tests of coagulation. Abnormalities of factor XIII are detected in clot solubility tests only. Some characteristics of fibrinogen and factor XIII are shown in Table 6.4.

The overall scheme of coagulation is shown in Figure 6.10.

Six of the eight proteins involved in the production of fibrin are activated during the coagulation sequence, and the other two (VIII and V) are cofactors of this activation. Each of the six proteins circulates as an inactive enzyme precursor and activation releases a proteolytic enzyme.

Table 6.3 Coagulation factors of the extrinsic and common pathway

Factor	MW	Plasma concentration, μg/ml	Plasma half life	Site of synthesis	Adsorbed by
VII	63 000	2	2–6 hrs	liver Vit. K. dependent	BaSO$_4$, Al(OH)$_3$
X	55 000	6–8	1–2 d	liver Vit. K. dependent	BaSO$_4$, Al(OH)$_3$
V	290 000	?	12–16 hrs	liver	—
prothrom-bin	72 000	200	2–3 d	liver Vit. K. dependent	BaSO$_4$, AL(OH)$_3$

Table 6.4   Fibrinogen and Factor XIII

Factor	MW	Plasma concentration, g/l	Plasma half life	Site of synthesis
fibrinogen	340 000	1·5–4·0	4–5 d	liver
factor XIII	320 000	?	3–7 d	liver megakaryocytes

Natural inhibitors of coagulation

Uncontrolled action of these proteolytic enzymes, which could lead to generalized intravascular clotting, is prevented by plasma protease inhibitors. These are plasma proteins that inhibit and neutralize a wide variety of proteolytic enzymes. At least four may play a role in coagulation, viz α_2 macroglobulin, antithrombin III, α_1 antitrypsin and C_1 inactivator.

Antithrombin III, also called heparin cofactor or antiXa, is probably the main plasma antagonist of thrombin, activated factor X, factor IX and factor XI. Its neutralizing action is greatly potentiated and accelerated by heparin. The interaction between antithrombin III and small amounts of heparin is the basis of low dose heparin prophylaxis for venous thrombosis.

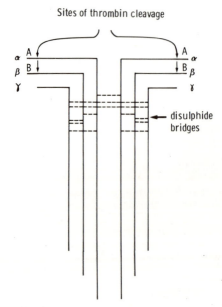

Fig. 6.8 Fibrinogen molecule.

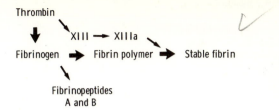

Fig. 6.9 Formation of stable fibrin.

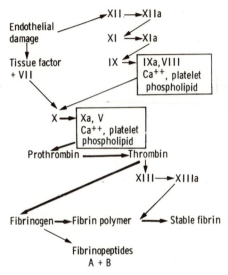

Fig. 6.10 The overall coagulation sequence.

Fibrinolysis

The dissolution of fibrin deposits *in vivo* or fibrin clots *in vitro* is called fibrinolysis. It is caused by a proteolytic enzyme in plasma called plasmin released by the activation of the fibrinolytic system. The components of the fibrinolytic system are plasminogen activators, plasminogen, as well as inhibitors of activation and/or plasmin, as shown schematically in Figure 6.11.

Plasminogen is a protein present in plasma in a concentration of 0.1–0.2 g/l. It is synthesized in liver and probably in bone marrow eosinophils. Plasminogen activators are proteolytic enzymes converting plasminogen into plasmin, and are present in plasma, urine (as a peptide called urokinase) and in cells such as endothelial cells, platelets and leucocytes. Plasminogen can also be activated by streptokinase, a peptide produced by haemolytic streptococci. Human plasminogen

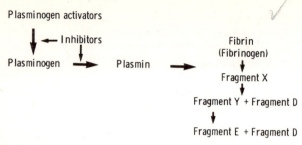

Fig. 6.11 Fibrinolysis.

and plasmin form a complex with streptokinase which acts as activator of plasminogen. If excess streptokinase is added all plasminogen is complexed with streptokinase and no plasmin can be generated.

Plasmin opens peptide linkages in both fibrinogen and fibrin and many different fragments are formed. The larger molecular weight fragments are grouped according to molecular weight into fragments X, Y, D and E. The largest fragments, X, are clotted by thrombin and are incorporated into fibrin clots. The Y fragments have anticoagulant effects due to interference with fibrin polymerization. Fragments D and E are the derivatives commonly found in the plasma of patients with disseminated intravascular coagulation. Fibrinogen degradation products are rapidly cleared from the circulation by the liver and by the mononuclear-phagocytic cell system in general.

An increase in the activity of plasminogen activators in plasma is often demonstrated by laboratory tests, but a measurable increase in free plasmin rarely follows because antiplasmin (inhibitory) systems neutralize plasmin generated from plasminogen. Antithrombin III, α_2 macroglobulin, α_1 antitrypsin and C1 inactivator can slowly neutralize plasmin. Immediate neutralization is provided by a highly specific fast antiplasmin. In contrast, plasmin arises readily in thrombi. To explain this, two hypothesis are proposed: one, that in the thrombus plasminogen is activated in close proximity to fibrin and acts before the inhibitors can interfere. The other hypothesis suggests that the plasmin is formed in the circulation and rapidly complexes with inhibitors, mainly α_2 macroglobulin. When these complexes come into contact with a thrombus, plasmin is dissociated and acts on fibrin, whereas α_2 macroglobulin is excluded from the fibrin mesh due to its high molecular weight.

Interaction of coagulation, fibrinolysis and kinin formation
The three systems are linked through factor XII. Factor XII can be activated by either of two mechanisms; contact with a negatively

charged surface, such as glass, kaolin or collagen, or proteolysis by enzymes such as plasmin, kallikrein or factor XIa. Factor XIIa in turn activates factor XI (coagulation), plasminogen activator (fibrinolysis) and prekallikrein (kallikrein-kinin system). Kinins are peptides that mediate the inflammatory reaction, especially vascular permeability, leukocyte migration and pain production. The simplified scheme of these interactions is shown on Fig. 6.12.

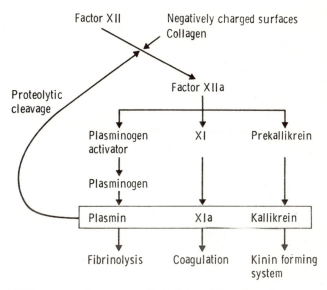

Fig. 6.12 Interaction of coagulation, fibrinolysis and kinin formation.

In the injured blood vessel, factor XII is activated through contact with exposed collagen. This 'surface activated' factor XII activates the coagulation, fibrinolytic and kinin-forming sequences. Enzymes from the three systems in turn cleave the remaining factor XII into more factor XIIa, thus amplifying all the reactions.

Investigation of haemostasis

Tests of vascular function
Tests which assess vascular function are the bleeding time and the capillary resistance test. The *bleeding time* consists of making a small puncture through the skin and noting the time required for bleeding to stop. Three methods of puncturing the skin are commonly used: Duke's method, Ivy's method (both using sterile lancets) and a method that uses a specifically designed blade, Mielke's template. The last method is the most sensitive of the three.

The capillary resistance test (Hess's test) consists of inflating a sphygmomanometer cuff around the arm and inspecting the forearm for small punctate haemorrhages after a period of inflation.

These tests are also abnormal if platelets are abnormal in numbers or function.

Platelet function tests

A low platelet count or abnormally functioning platelets produce a prolonged bleeding time and a positive capillary resistance test.

Platelet aggregation in vitro is measured by the change in light transmission of platelet-rich plasma after the addition of an aggregating agent. More light is transmitted as the platelets clump. A normal tracing is shown in Figure 6.13. The primary wave is absent in thrombasthenia, whereas there is absence of the secondary wave after taking aspirin and many anti-inflammatory drugs as well as in a platelet disorder called storage pool disease.

Platelet retention on glass beads. When anticoagulated or fresh blood samples are passed through a small column of glass beads a proportion of platelets is retained on the glass surface. Platelet retention or adhesiveness is affected by the properties of platelets themselves, packed cell volume and plasma proteins. Platelet retention is reduced or absent in thrombasthenia, some cases of von Willebrand's disease, uraemia, scurvy and many other conditions. Increased platelet

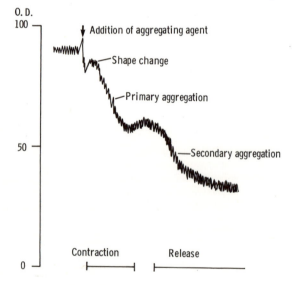

Fig. 6.13 Normal platelet aggregation.

adhesiveness to glass is sometimes demonstrated in arterial or venous disease and after surgery.

Platelet factor 3 availability. This test measures the clot-promoting activity of platelets provided by platelet phospholipid or PF_3. The kaolin-cephalin time is measured on mixtures of platelet rich and platelet poor plasma from patient and control. PF_3 availability is abnormal in thrombasthenia, in uraemia, myeloma and myelo-proliferative disorders.

Platelet nucleotide content. The content of platelet nucleotides is sometimes measured to establish the diagnosis of storage pool disease where platelet ADP and ATP are reduced or absent.

Tests for platelet antibodies. Techniques for demonstration of platelet antibodies are described in Chapter 7.

Blood coagulation tests

In general whole blood or plasma from the patient is allowed to clot in the presence of calcium ions and various other reagents and the time taken for the sample to clot is compared with a normal control blood or plasma in the same system. The screening tests commonly used are the whole blood clotting time, kaolin-cephalin time, prothrombin time, thrombin time and prothrombin consumption test.

Whole blood clotting time. Venous blood is placed into a new glass tube and allowed to clot at $37°C$. Normal blood takes usually between 5 and 10 minutes to clot. Normal whole blood clotting time excludes a gross deficiency in the intrinsic pathway and coagulation sequence in general, but will not detect milder defects which may nevertheless cause severe bleeding.

Kaolin-cephalin time is carried out by mixing the patients plasma with kaolin, brain extract (cephalin) and calcium and allowing it to clot. The normal range depends on the reagents used and is usually between 30 and 40 seconds. Kaolin-cephalin time is an overall test of clotting function and reduced levels of any of the clotting factors (fibrinogen, prothrombin, V, VIII, IX, X, XI and XII will be reflected in the prolonged clotting time. However, increased concentration or activation of one or more individual factors may mask a deficiency of another factor, and in bleeding patients further investigation is necessary even if this test is within the normal range.

One stage-prothrombin time. This test is carried out by mixing plasma, thromboplastin (brain extract) and calcium. Normal plasma will clot in 11–14 seconds, depending on the thromboplastin used. It is sensitive to reduced levels of factor V, VII, X, prothrombin and fibrinogen. It is extensively used to control anticoagulant treatment.

Prothrombin consumption test. This test is carried out on plasma and serum. Calcium is added to both and at given time intervals aliquots subsampled into tubes containing fibrinogen, and the time for fibrinogen to clot recorded. When haemostasis is normal, plasma will clot fibrinogen very rapidly (in 12–20 seconds), whereas serum takes two to three minutes or more. The results are expressed as the plasma time over serum time × 100 and normal values are less than 20 per cent. Such low values indicate that coagulation was efficient and that serum contains little remaining prothrombin. If haemostasis is inefficient more prothrombin remains in the serum, giving shorter serum times and a higher percentage. The test is sensitive to deficiencies of all coagulation factors and to platelet malfunction and may occasionally be the only positive screening test in minor defects of coagulation.

Calcium thrombin time. This test is carried out by adding a mixture of calcium and thrombin to patient's plasma. Depending on the concentration of thrombin, normal plasma will clot in 10–20 seconds. The test is prolonged when fibrinogen levels are low, fibrinogen is abnormal or when high concentrations of fibrin degradation products (FDP) are present.

Further investigation consists in performing coagulation factor assays (factor VIII, IX, X, VII, V, XI and XII and prothrombin), fibrinogen estimation, clot solubility testing, measurement of inhibitors and various immunological techniques. These tests can detect even a minor deficiency of a single factor when used with suitable standards in a laboratory with technical expertise.

The results of coagulation factor assays are expressed as percentages of normal pooled plasma. In the case of factor VIII the results are expressed as international units per dl. calculated by comparison to a freeze dried pooled plasma, for example the British Standard for factor VIII in the UK. With all factors, values below 40 per cent (4 iu/dl for factor VIII) are abnormally low, and indicate a deficiency either congenital or acquired as in liver disease.

Tests of fibrinolysis

Tests of fibrinolytic activity are largely qualitative and the significance of minor changes are uncertain. The only congenital abnormality recognized is the congenital deficiency of the fast antiplasmin.

Plasminogen activator. The levels of plasminogen activator are measured by dilute whole blood clot lysis time or euglobulin lysis in tubes or on a fibrin plate. The principle is to remove natural inhibitors of plasminogen activation by dilution (whole blood clot lysis time) or acid pH (euglobulin lysis) and to record the time taken to lyse a blood or plasma clot. Generally a dilute whole blood clot lyses in 2–6 hours and the euglobulin lysis time is between 30 minutes and 300 minutes. Very short lysis times are found in the presence of brisk fibrinolysis, whether due to stress, strenuous exercise, venous occlusion, or as a response to disseminated intravascular fibrin deposition. Prolonged lysis time is found in patients with vascular disease, obese individuals, sometimes after surgery or trauma and in many other conditions.

Plasminogen can be measured by its action in the proteolytic breakdown of casein after activation by streptokinase or urokinase. This technique is rarely used for investigation of patients.

Fibrin-fibrinogen degradation products can be measured by a variety of techniques, mostly immunological or radioimmunometric. Fragments X, Y, D and E have antigenic determinants common to fibrinogen and thus react with fibrinogen antisera. If the serum sample tested contains FDP, the fibrinogen antiserum will be neutralized during the incubation time and hence there will be no agglutination of fibrinogen coated Latex particles or tanned red cells. FDP concentration is expressed as μg/ml. Normal serum generally contains less than 10 μg/ml. Slightly elevated values are found commonly in liver disease, septicaemia, eclampsia, thromboembolic disease, myeloproliferative disorders and after surgery. Very high levels of FDP (over 600 μg/ml) are usually found in fulminant disseminated intravascular coagulation.

Paracoagulation tests. If plasma contains complexes of fibrin monomers with fibrinogen or FDP, these complexes will give rise to a transparent gel in the presence of ethanol or protamine sulphate. This phenomenon is called paracoagulation. Positive paracoagulation tests are found in many diseases including pneumonia and septicaemia and are of importance only if accompanied by abnormalities of fibrinogen or increased levels of FDP.

References

Alkajaersig N, Fletcher A P, Sherry S 1959 The mechanism of clot dissolution by plasmin. Journal Clinical Investigation 38: 1086–1095

Ambrus C M, Markus G 1960 Plasmin-antiplasmin complex as a reservoir of fibrinolytic enzyme. American Journal Physiology 199: 491–494

Barrowcliffe T W, Johnson E A, Thomas D H 1978 Antithrombin III and heparin. British Medical Bulletin 34: 143–150

Baugh R F, Houghie C 1979 The chemistry of blood coagulation. Clinics in Haematology 8: 3–30

Bloom A L, Peake I R 1977 Factor VIII and its inherited disorders. British Medical Bulletin 33: 219–224

Collen D 1976 Identification and some properties of a new fast reacting plasmin inhibitor in human plasma. European Journal Biochemistry 69: 209–216

Curtis C G, Lorand L 1977 The fibrin-stabilizing system of plasma. In:
    Haemostasis: Biochemistry. Physiology and Pathology, Ogston D, Bennett B eds
    p 186–201, John Wiley and Sons, London
Kernoff P B A, McNicol G P 1977 Normal and abnormal fibrinolysis. British
    Medical Bulletin 33: 239–244
Moncada S, Vane J R 1978 Unstable metabolites of arachidonic acid. British
    Medical Bulletin 34: 129–136
Ogston D, Bennett B 1978 Surface mediated reactions in the formation of
    thrombin, plasmin and kallikrein. British Medical Bulletin 34: 107–112
Sixma J J, Wester J 1977 The haemostatic plug. Seminars in Haematology 14:
    265–300

7

Immune mechanisms

The mechanisms that protect an individual against infective agents may be non-specific (innate immunity) or be specific against the particular agent. The non-specific agencies include lining squamous and epithelial surfaces of the body and the inhibitory effect on bacterial growth of secretions on these surfaces. If this barrier is penetrated, phagocytosis occurs aided by bactericidal substances such as lysozyme and the action of complement activated through the alternate pathway. Within the cell interferon may inhibit replication of viral agents.

The specific mechanisms involve the production of antibodies and the deployment of complex cellular changes.

The humoral antibody response
Infection with an organism such as a streptococcus is followed by the appearance in blood of antibodies specifically reacting with this bacterium and its products. Following the first contact with the organism there is a relatively slow rise in the level of serum antibody reaching a peak in the third week followed by a fall. This is the primary response. A second infection with the same organism however is followed by a more rapid appearance of antibody produced in greater amount. This is the secondary response.

The lymphocyte is the cell central to these responses. It is now believed that each lymphocyte can make only one antibody and molecules of that antibody are part of the cell-surface receptors of the lymphocyte. Bacteria (the antigen) will combine with those lymphocytes whose surface antibody provides a good fit. This fit is determined by the physical and chemical configuration of antigen and antibody and forms the basis of specificity. The factors concerned are electrostatic charges such as positively charged amino groups (NH_3^+) and negatively charged carboxyl $(COO-)$ groups linking antigen and antibody, formation of hydrogen bridges between hydrophylic groups, as well as attachment of water repellent surfaces or hydrophobic groups. When an antigen has found a lymphocyte with a good fit, that lymphocyte is stimulated to divide and so give rise to a clone of cells all making antibody of the same specificity. The initial cell is a small lymphocyte, those that divide become large lymphocytes. Some of the latter revert to small lymphocytes, become memory cells and are available years later to initiate a secondary response. The primary response is concerned with the establishment of a new clone of antibody-secreting cells (these are morphologically plasma cells). At a second appearance, the organism encounters a larger population of lymphocytes with the appropriate antibody and a correspondingly more rapid response ensues. The lymphocytes carrying antibody on their surface are called B-lymphocytes and the demonstration of such surface antibody by immunofluorescent techniques is the method used for identification. In chicks the development of normal B-lymphocytes requires the presence of a lymphoid organ (Bursa of Fabricius). In man, haemopoietic tissue such as marrow serves a similar role.

The early response to infection is the production of IgM antibodies but this declines rapidly and IgG immunoglobin replaces it reaching a maximum over a longer period and secretion often continues over many years. A humoral response to an antigen leading to the production of a clone of antibody-secreting lymphocytes also requires the cooperation of another type of lymphocyte called a T-lymphocyte and of a macrophage.

T-lymphocytes are lymphocytes that have been processed by or are in some way dependent on, the thymus gland. They are concerned with cell-mediated immunity. Human T-cells react with sheep red blood cells so that they come to form a ring or rosette around the lymphocyte and this is the usual way they are identified.

Humoral responses may be considerably depressed if the thymus gland is removed shortly after birth. The T-cell, which itself cannot make antibody, cooperates with B-lymphocytes and help them to develop into antibody-forming cells. This role has been called a helper role and these T-lymphocytes helper cells.

The antibody response will also fail to occur if mononuclear cells (macrophages or monocytes) are removed. It has been suggested that antigen is altered and concentrated on the macrophage surface and presented to the lymphocyte in an optimal manner.

The antibodies (immunoglobulins)
The humoral antibodies synthesized by the plasma cells have a common basic structure (Fig. 7.1). Each molecule is made up of four

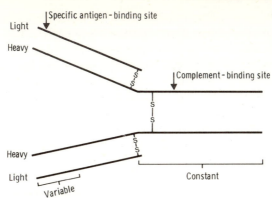

Fig. 7.1 The immunoglobulin molecule.

peptide chains, the longer ones termed heavy chains and the short ones light chains, all joined by disulphide bonds as shown in the figure. The variable (or N-terminal) end of the light and heavy chains is the portion of the antibody that reacts with the antigen and carries the configuration that determines the antibody specificity. Within each immunoglobulin class the remainder of the molecule is relatively constant in structure.

Treatment of IgG with proteolytic enzymes splits the molecule. Papain produces breaks of the heavy chains between the S–S linkages so that three fragments ensue. Two are identical (part of the heavy chain and light chain), combine with antibody and have been called Fab (fragment antigen binding). The third is the remains of the heavy chains, does not combine with antigen and is called the Fc (fragment crystallizable) fragment. Pepsin splits the heavy chain in the Fc region beyond the SS link leaving a large fragment that can react bivalently with antigen.

Myeloma is a disease due to proliferation of a single clone of plasma cells. The myeloma cells in any one patient synthesize and release a single uniform immunoglobulin or portion of an immunoglobulin. Specific antisera have been produced against these myeloma proteins and their use have enabled us to divide the immunoglobulins into various types.

Light chains. The light chains of the immunoglobulin molecule are serologically of two types termed kappa (κ) or lambda (λ). One of the proteins that may appear in the urine in myeloma (Bence-Jones protein) is the light chain portion of the immunoglobulin molecule and likewise is either kappa or lambda in type.

Heavy chains. In addition to characterizing the light chains, antisera against the heavy chains make it possible to divide antibodies into major immunoglobulin groups termed immunoglobulin-G or IgG, IgA, IgM, IgD and IgE.

Whereas the variable portions of the heavy and light chains are concerned with the specificity of the antibody, the Fc part of the heavy chain is concerned with its biological activity, that is, its distribution in the body, passage across the placenta, fixation of complement etc.

Small differences in the structure of the heavy chains have made it possible to subdivide IgG immunoglobulins into four subclasses (IgG1 to IgG4) and IgA and IgM into two subclasses.

IgG constitutes about 80 per cent of the serum immunoglobulin, IgA 13 per cent and IgM 6 per cent. IgD and IgE are present in only very small amounts. IgG and IgM bind complement. Only IgG immunoglobulins cross the placenta to reach the fetus and this 'passive' transfer of antibodies provides protection for the newborn in the early months of life.

IgA is primarily the immunoglobulin of secretory tissues particularly the gastrointestinal tract. It is produced by plasma cells within the secretory organ such as stomach and lamina propria of the small gut. Usually two molecules join to form a dimer and an additional structure called an end piece produced by epithelial cells is attached to the dimer.

The immunoglobulin unit has a MW between 150000 and 200000. IgM consists of five immunoglobulin units (MW 900000). Because of the multiple binding sites for antigen on IgM molecules, IgM is a potent agglutinin, the best example being cold antibodies which may cause haemolytic anaemia. Naturally acquired agglutinins like anti-A and anti-B are also mainly IgM in type.

IgE is concerned with allergic-type reactions. IgE, but also IgG, attach to mast cells and a reaction of these surface antibodies with the antigen causes a degranulation of the contents of the large basophilic granules with a release of their histamine. Contact of an antigen with IgE in the bronchial tree gives rise to bronchospasm and symptoms of asthma.

T- B- and null cells

Uncommitted lymphocytes probably arising in the marrow are modified in the marrow in man (B-cell) or in the thymus gland (T-cell). Some 70 per cent of blood lymphocytes are T-cells 10–20 per cent B-cells and the remainder so-called null cells.

Immunoglobulins are present on the surface of the B-lymphocyte. Most cells have IgD and IgM but some react with the Fc portion from

IgG. If the immunoglobulin in the cell surface is removed by a proteolytic enzyme, fresh immunoglobulin is synthesized over the next few hours. The immunoglobulin is thought to be present in the free state in the plasma membrane of the cell and may be agglutinated into patches by anti-IgG or even form a cap at one end of the cell. Morphologically the B-cells develop into plasma cells. Within lymph glands B-cells are aggregated in the cortical lymphoid follicles.

In the lymph gland T-cell areas lie between the hilum and cortex. T-lymphocytes have a role as helper cell in the humoral response. They are responsible for a number of reactions which while retaining the antigenic specificity associated with humoral reactions, are nevertheless not due to surface immunoglobulins but to cellular mechanisms. These reactions are termed cell-mediated immunity and an example is the skin reaction produced by the intradermal injection of a product of the tubercle bacillus called the Mantoux reaction. A positive reaction in the skin consists of a raised area of induration at the site of injection reaching a maximum 48 hours later and associated with considerable macrophage infiltration. A cell-mediated response occurs as the usual reaction to many viruses, fungi (candida) and bacteria (tubercle), contact dermatitis and in rejection of a transplanted organ. Loss of the thymus gland in early life results in impaired cell-mediated immunity. The way in which the T-cell recognizes an antigen is not known but there are receptors on the cell which are not immunoglobulins. So called killer T-cells are those which exert a cytotoxic effect on a genetically dissimilar graft from a member of the same species but many K cells are null-cells.

A further population of T-cells are concerned with regulation of B-cell responses and these have been termed suppressor cells. Finally T-cells may release substances—lymphokines which may attract macrophages to the site of a reaction.

When the number of B- and T-cells in a blood sample have been counted the total may fall short of 100 per cent. The remainder may be termed null cells. Among these are cells with killer functions as well as haemopoietic stem cells.

The activity of B-lymphocytes in man is gauged by measuring serum immunoglobulin levels which are normally

serum IgG   0·8 to 1·6 g/100 ml
serum IgA   0·14 to 0·4 g/100 ml
serum IgM   0·05 to 0·2 g/100 ml

B-lymphocyte responses are also measured by noting whether the subject can produce serum antibodies following antigenic stimulation, e.g. injection of pneumococcal polysaccharide.

Specific T-cell activity, that is, a reaction occurring when sensitized T-lymphocytes react with an antigen, is detected by:

1. *Migration inhibition test.* White blood cells are concentrated from a fresh blood sample and taken up in a capillary tube. When the capillary is placed in medium in a chamber the leucocytes and macrophages will migrate out of the end of the tube as illustrated in Figure 7.2. If an antigen which the T-cells recognize is present in the fluid in the chamber, soluble substances are released which will prevent the cellular migration (Fig. 7.3). The substance has been termed migration inhibition factor (MIF).

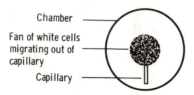

Fig. 7.2 Neutrophils and macrophages migrating out of a capillary tube into culture medium.

2. *Transformation.* The sensitized T-cells, like the B-cells, on contact with antigen (or antigen-antibody complex) undergo cell division and this can be used as a test for cell-mediated immunity. When cell division occurs ^{14}C-thymidine (added to the medium) will be incorporated into the nuclear material of the new cells.

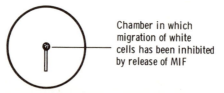

Fig. 7.3 Inhibition of migration of white cells into the medium (compare Fig. 7.2) following release of migration inhibition factor by T-lymphocytes which have 'reacted' with an antigen in the culture medium.

3. *Dinitrochlorobenzene* (DNCB) when applied to the skin, stimulates cell-mediated immunity in man. When a further dose of DNCB is applied a week later a typical skin response occurs 48 hours later due to newly sensitized T-lymphocytes.
4. *Tuberculin test.* A positive skin test to a product of the tubercle bacillus (tuberculin or purified protein derivative—PPD) is evidence of specific T-cell activity to this antigen.

Antigen-antibody reactions

Humoral antibody combines with antigen. Each molecule of IgG and IgA can bind with two units of antigen but IgM can bind five or possibly ten antigen units. The better the fit between antigen and antibody the higher the antibody affinity for the antigen.

In vitro an antigen-antibody reaction may culminate in:

1. *Precipitation*, that is, the antigen-antibody complex comes out of solution. If the reaction occurs in a diffusable medium such as agar, the precipitate will occur at a line where the most favourable concentrations of the 2 reagents meet (Fig. 7.4).
2. *Agglutination*. Bacteria or red blood cells may be clumped together as a result of cross linking by multivalent antibody.
3. *Antiglobulin Reaction*. Red blood cells may react with an antibody without any obvious change in these cells. However, if a further antibody (an antiglobulin) which reacts with the immunoglobin on the red cell surface is added, agglutination occurs (Fig. 7.5).
4. *Immunofluorescence*. Similarly, if the antiglobulin is conjugated with a fluorescent dye, this too will attach to immunoglobin on the cell or bacterial surface and render such a cell bearing antibody, visible in ultra-violet light with an appropriate microscope.

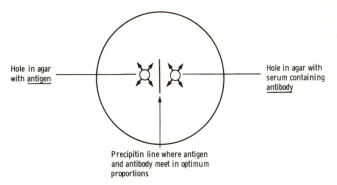

Hole in agar with <u>antigen</u>

Hole in agar with serum containing <u>antibody</u>

Precipitin line where antigen and antibody meet in *optimum* proportions

Fig. 7.4 Antigen and antibody have been placed in two wells in an agar medium. Both diffuse out into the medium. At a certain concentration of each of these reagents the immune complex (antigen-antibody) is precipitated to form a visible line.

5. *Complement-Fixation*. Complement is a complex series of at least nine protein components which react in sequence with an antigen-antibody complex. The reactions can lead to damage to the cell surface and in the case of red cells, to haemolysis. The fixation

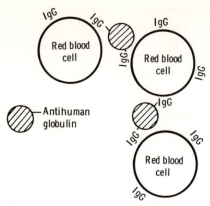

Fig. 7.5 Antiglobulin molecules can cross link between antibody on the surface of two red cells and so produce agglutination seen with the naked eye.

of complement by an antigen-antibody complex may be used as evidence that an antigen-antibody reaction has occurred. Thus antigen and antibody are allowed to react and complement (for example in guinea-pig serum) added (Fig. 7.6A). The antigen-antibody complex will react with all the complement. When sheep red cells sensitized with antibody (haemolysin) are added there is

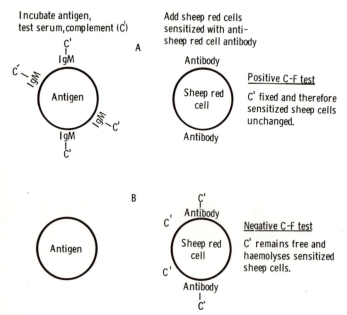

Fig. 7.6 The complement-fixation test.

no surplus complement available to produce haemolysis. This is a positive reaction. If however, no antibody was available in the initial mixture, free complement will be present (Fig. 7.6B) which can now react with the sensitized sheep cells and which will undergo haemolysis. This is a negative result.

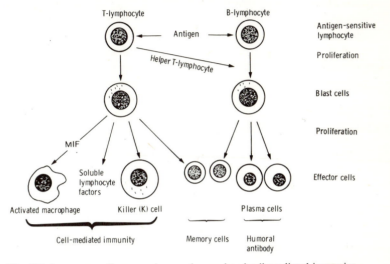

Fig. 7.7 A summary of current views on humoral and cell-mediated immunity.

In vivo reaction of an antibody and complement with invading bacteria may itself be lethal to the bacterium and it facilitates phagocytosis by neutrophils and macrophages. The presence of both humoral and cell-mediated immunity enables the host to overcome and resist subsequent infection with many bacterial and viral infections.

Figure 7.7 summarizes current views on the role of lymphocytes in humoral and cell-mediated immunity.

Complement
The effects ascribed to complement result from a sequence of reactions between serum proteins present in plasma. The sequence of reactions is initiated by the presence of the complex formed when antigen and antibody have reacted, that is, an immune complex. However the sequence can be triggered off by agents other than immune complexes including bacterial endotoxin and snake venoms and this has been termed the alternate pathway. The reaction involves an immune complex with either IgM or IgG and complement C1q which binds to

a receptor on the Fc portion of the immunoglobulin molecule. Two further components bind and these are C1r and C1s. The latter then functions as an esterase enzyme which activates further proteins in the sequence (C_4 and C_2). The complex is now able to split C_3 into two fractions (C_3a and C_3b). The alternate path bypasses the earlier phases acting directly on C_3. The products of C_3 cleavage are chemotactic for leucocytes and promote adherence of the affected cell to polymorphs and macrophages (immune adherence). Involvement of further complement components (C_5 to C_9) produce damage of cell membranes and in the case of the red cell bearing IgM or IgG, holes are produced which cause the haemoglobin to leak out (haemolysis).

Reference

Roit I M 1977 Essential immunology. Blackwell, Oxford

8

Some human antigens and their inheritance

The nuclei of human cells have 46 chromosomes, that is 23 pairs (diploid state). All inherited characteristics are present in genes which are sited on particular parts of the chromosome. Each site is called a locus and each inherited characteristic is present on the same locus on both of the paired chromosomes. The ova produced in the ovary and the spermatozoa produced in the testis contain 23 single chromosomes (haploid state) and their fusion reunites the 23 pairs.

The two genes on the loci on a pair of chromosomes may be the same (homozygous) or they may be different (heterozygous). Where a number of alternate genes exist for a single locus they are called allelomorphic genes or alleles. The genes present in an individual constitute the genotype. All these genes cannot always be detected; only some are manifest and these that can be detected make up the phenotype. Thus testing red cells may show them to be of group A (phenotype) but the genes present are either AA or AO (genotype).

A different situation pertains in relation to the sex chromosomes. Sexual characteristics are carried on chromosomes termed X and Y. Females have a pair of X chromosomes (XX); males have X and Y (XY). In meiosis (segregation of chromosomes into sex cells) ova each have a single X chromosome. In the male the sperm has either an X or a Y chromosome—an X sperm fertilizing the ovum (XX) produces a female offspring; a Y sperm fertilizing the ovum (XY) produces a male offspring. The X and Y chromosomes are unequal in size, the X being larger. Thus more chromatin is present in female cells (XX) than in male cells (XY) and this is seen on inspection of the cells in the form of the drumstick attached to the nucleus of neutrophil polymorphs in females or the Barr body, an extra piece of chromatin on the edge of the nucleus of cells from other tissues such as skin.

Whether a gene is expressed or not depends on whether it is dominant or recessive. If there is a dominant gene on one locus and a recessive on the other, only the dominant will be expressed. A recessive characteristic will only be expressed clinically if it is present on both chromosomes, that is, in the homozygous state. However, the biochemical effect of the presence of 2, 1 or 0 genes for a particular activity can be measured. Thus the vitamin B_{12} carrier protein, Transcobalamin II is transmitted as an autosomal gene. When one abnormal gene is present the subject has half the level of carrier protein than those siblings who have 2 normal genes. When the subject has 2 abnormal genes there is no carrier protein and he has a severe megaloblastic anaemia. Similar data have been accumulated in relation to many enzymes in man. The situation is different in relation to those characteristics transmitted on that part of the X chromosome (hatched in Figure 8.1), that is not matched by the Y chromosome in males. All genes on that hatched part of the X chromosome are expressed in males, but recessive genes will only be expressed in females if present on both X chromosomes. Genes controlling the level of anti-haemophilic globulin (factor VIII) and the enzyme, glucose-6-phosphate dehydrogenase, are carried on this part of the X chromosome. Diseases due to abnormalities of these genes (haemophilia and haemolytic anaemia) are transmitted by females but manifest in males, who are genetically hemizygous.

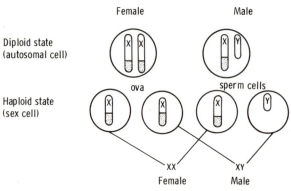

Fig. 8.1 X and Y chromosomes in sex determination. Genes located on the hatched portion of the X chromosome are expressed in males. Genes controlling factor VIII levels and glucose-6-phosphate dehydrogenase are located here.

In females only one of the X chromosomes in each cell is expressed and the effects of the second are inactivated. This inactivation of one of the two X chromosomes in each cell in females is called the Lyon hypothesis. In relation to heterozygotes for glucose-6-phosphate dehydrogenase deficiency, either the X chromosome with the normal gene remains active (when that cell will have normal enzyme activity) or the other X chromosome with a gene producing a defective enzyme remains active when G6PD activity will be very low. In females heterozygous for G6PD deficiency half the red blood cells, in fact, have normal enzyme activity and the other half very low activity as expected on the Lyon hypothesis.

The inheritance of many characters in man have been studied particularly those that can be measured in a blood sample. These include plasma components such as haptoglobins, transferrins, lipoproteins, immunoglobulins, and alkaline phosphatase. In red cells, antigens that have been studied include blood groups, haemoglobins and red cell enzymes. White blood cell antigens have been studied in relation to tissue typing.

Blood group antigens

More than 400 antigens can be recognized on the surface of human red blood cells. The more important systems include ABO, Rhesus, MNS, I, P, Lewis, Lutheran, Kell, Duffy, Kidd and Xg.

ABO blood group system

Antigens of the ABO system

The antigens A and B may be present singly or together (AB). The absence of both antigens gives group O. The genes are inherited as dominant characteristics, that is, when the gene is present the antigen is expressed (Table 8.1).

Table 8.1 ABO System

	Group	Frequency %	Antibody
A	A_1	34·8	anti-B
	A_2	9·9	
B		8·6	anti-A
AB	A_1B	2·6	no antibody
	A_2B	0·6	
O		43·5	anti-A + anti-B

The A antigen is subgrouped into A_1 and the weaker antigen A_2. The A_2 antigen in red cells is complicated by the presence in serum of anti-A_1 in 2 per cent of A_2 persons and in 20 per cent of A_2B persons. Group A_2 red cells may have only a quarter of the antigenic sites on the red cell surface present in A_1 red cells, but there may also be a qualitative difference.

The ABO as well as Lewis antigens are glycoproteins consisting of a peptide of 15 amino acids followed by the sequence of carbohydrate residues shown in Figure 8.2. The product of the H gene leads to an addition of a fucose residue to the H antigen. Further additions controlled by the appropriate genes give rise to A, B and Lewis substance. In group O the H antigen remains unaltered.

In the rare 'Bombay' group the H gene is replaced by the recessive allele h which fails to convert precursor substance to H antigen. As H antigen is lacking neither A nor B antigen can be formed although A

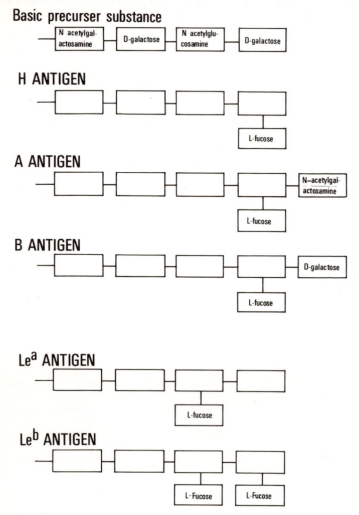

Fig. 8.2 Structure of A, B, H and Lewis substances.

and B genes may be present. These cells are called Oh. The serum of an Oh individual contains anti-A+anti-B+anti-H and is therefore incompatible with all blood except that of another Oh donor.

A, B and H antigens are present in the red cell membrane as well as in most body cells including white cells and platelets. These antigens are also present in water soluble form in tissues and in most of the body fluids of the 80 per cent of the population who possess secretor genes. These soluble antigens or blood group specific substances are present in plasma, saliva, meconium, semen, urine, gastric juice, sweat, tears and bile, but not in cerebrospinal fluid. The ABO antigens are stable and their detection on dried blood stains and other fluids is used in forensic serology. They can still be isolated in Egyptian and Japenese mummies.

A_3. The presence of the rare allelic gene A_3 is detected by very characteristic weak reactions with anti-A and anti-A+B showing very clear small clumps in a sea of free cells. In an AB individual the A_2 antigen is frequently weakened in the presence of B antigen. Thus family studies should be done before deciding that an individual has the A_3B rather than the A_2B blood group.

A_x. This is the term used for a group of weakly reacting A cells. Typically these show a very weak or absent reaction with anti-A but a clear reaction with anti A+B. Anti-A_2 is often present. Secretors show H substance only.

A_m. In this rare group the cells appear to be group O but there is no anti-A or anti-A_1 in serum. Saliva of secretors however, contains A and H substance and the cells can be shown to have weak A antigenicity using absorption-elution studies.

A int. The antigen strength of this group is between that of A_1 and A_2, and is often seen in Negro samples. The H antigen strength is greater than expected.

Weak B. Variants containing a weak B antigen are occasionally described.

Acquired B. This is a temporary gain of B-like antigen from intestinal bacteria, and may be associated with a colonic lesion such as a neoplasm in which there is necrosis. It occurs typically in A_1 individuals who show an apparent change of group to A_1B. This may also occur in group A_2.

Chimeras. These may give rise to an interesting ABO group anomaly. In dizygotic twins where the early red cell precursors have migrated between twins of differing ABO blood groups, there are two co-existing red cell populations. This gives a mixed blood picture. Tolerance occurs, and there is a lack of the expected antibody.

Antibodies of the ABO system

Naturally-occurring antibodies develop in the ABO system after the age of three months. The expected antibodies are absent in infants under three months, although cord blood may contain passively transferred maternal IgG antibody. Individuals with hypo- or agammaglobulinaemia lack these antibodies, and weaker antibodies are also seen in old age.

These naturally-acquired antibodies react best in the cold, and are primarily of IgM specificity. IgG and IgA components may also be present. Typically IgG anti-A occurs in group O people. Both IgM and IgG antibody may be haemolytic in character. IgG anti-A may occur in serum without known stimulus to anti-A production. However, antigenic stimulus may come from injection of vaccines containing A-like antigen, from transfusion of A cells or A group specific substance, or during pregnancy by a foeto-maternal bleed.

Anti A_1. This may be found in 2 per cent of A_2 and 20 per cent of A_2B persons as a naturally-occurring antibody. Where transfusion is required for such people, it is necessary to select A_2 donor blood. Although human anti-A_1 may be used for screening blood samples, the best reagent is a lectin prepared as a saline extract of the seeds of Dolichos biflorus which will only agglutinate A_1 cells.

Anti H. Pure anti-H is a rare antibody found only in the serum of individuals of the Oh 'Bombay' group. Lectins having this specificity may be prepared from seeds of Ulex europaeus or Lotus tetragonolobus, and are used for grouping samples for their H antigen content. A_1B and A_1 cells contain very little H antigen. O cells contain the maximum H antigen, and the other ABO groups show an intermediate range of activity.

An incomplete cold antibody is present in almost all normal human sera and attaches to red cells incubated at $4°C$ for more than two hours. This so-called normal incomplete cold antibody has an anti-H specificity which can be neutralised by H substance. The 'antibody' is not an immunoglobulin. The resulting cell coating is of complement. This phenomenon is a cause of false positive direct antiglobulin tests on clotted blood samples which have been refrigerated.

Anti-HI. Occasionally this antibody is found in the serum of A_1 or A_1B individuals. It has been called an anti-HI because it reacts with red cells having H as well as I antigens.

The Lewis system

Lewis antigens. The Lewis antigens occur primarily in body fluids and are adsorbed from the plasma on to the red cell. Unlike other blood group antigens they are not part of the red cell membrane. The antigens develop from the precursor of the ABH antigens, having differing terminal carbohydrate residues (Fig. 8.1). The development of Lewis antigens depends on the interaction of Lewis (*Le le*) Secretor (*Se se*) *Hh* and *ABO* genes (Table 8.6).

A person who has the Lewis gene (double or single dose) will convert precursor substance to Le^a substance. *Se* and *H* genes in double or single dose convert Le^a substance to Le^b substance giving the group $Le^{(a-b-)}$. In the absence of *Se* genes, the Le^a substance remains, giving the group $Le^{(a+b-)}$. When the *Le* genes are absent, the precursor substance is unaltered, and the group $Le^{(a-b-)}$ occurs. It is unaffected by *Se* and *H* genes.

Table 8.2   Lewis system

Lewis gene *Le*	Secretor gene *Se*	Red cell phenotype	Saliva and serum contain			Frequency %	
			Le^a	Le^b	ABH	Caucasian	Negroid
present	present	$Le^{(a-b+)}$	w	+	+	74	34
present	absent	$Le^{(a+b-)}$	+	−	−	23	19
absent	present	$Le^{(a-b-)}$	−	−	+	4	47

At birth the concentration of Lewis substance in plasma is very low, so that the red cell antigen is either absent or very weakly expressed. The correct Lewis group is obtained at about eighteen months of age.

Lewis antibodies. Lewis antibodies which are often naturally occurring, are IgM and will agglutinate cells more readily at room temperature than at 37°C. The antibodies bind complement, and may be detected using an indirect antiglobulin technique with a broad spectrum antiglobulin reagent.

Anti-Le^a is not uncommon, and many sera with anti-Le^a also contain anti-Le^b. For transfusion purposes $Le^{(a-b-)}$ blood must be given. Lewis antibodies occur in about 20 per cent of $Le^{(a-b-)}$ individuals, and this phenotype is found in four per cent of Caucasians and 47 per cent Negroes. These are a problem when blood transfusion is required, but do not complicate pregnancy as the IgM antibody does not cross the placenta.

The Rhesus system

The red cell antigens of the Rhesus system are the product of a complex of closely linked genes and are usually described in terms of three linked pairs of alleles. The main alleles are, Dd, Cc and Ee and the genes appear in this order on the chromosome. Other than d, each antigen is defined by a specific antibody. Antibody to d has not been encountered and d is defined as the absence of the D antigen. A symbol is used to represent different combinations of genes (Table 8.3).

Table 8.3 Rhesus nomenclature

CDE nomenclature	Short symbol
CDe	R^1
cDE	R^2
cDe	R^0
CDE	R^z
cde	r
Cde	r′
cdE	r″
CdE	r^

The term Rhesus Positive refers to the presence of the D antigen. Samples recorded as Rhesus Negative using anti-D only may possess the C or E antigen. Rhesus negative donor blood is C, D and E negative. Thus donors may be encountered who donate as 'Rh Positive' yet are negative with anti-D. These belong to the groups r′ or r″ and should be treated as Rh negative for transfusion or antenatal purposes. The more common combination of antigens are shown in Table 8.4.

Since no anti-d is available, Rhesus genotyping results are expressed as the 'Rhesus phenotype' giving the results of tests with specific antisera, and 'probable Rhesus genotype' which is an assessment of the probable antigen combination based on statistics.

Rarely, Rhesus-D Positive people have been found to have anti-D in their serum. They have only part of the D antigen, and possess an antibody to that part of the D antigen they lack.

D^u *Antigens.* The term D^u is used for a series of antigens giving some but not all of the reactions of the D antigen. The D^u antigens may be graded from 'low grade' to 'high grade'. High grade D^u examples are agglutinated by most anti-D sera. Low grade D^u samples are detected by few sera, and an enzyme or indirect antiglobulin technique is required. It is for this reason that in standard Rhesus grouping, two anti-D sera are used, and apparent D negative samples are checked using the indirect antiglobulin technique. D^u is suspected when differing Rh groups have been reported for a patient by different laboratories.

Table 8.4   Rhesus system

CDE nomenclature	Short symbol	Frequency in Caucasians %
CDe/cde	R_1r	32
CDe/CDe	R_1R_1	17
cde/cde	rr	15
CDe/cDE	R_1R_2	14
cDE/cde	R_2r	13
cDE/cDE	R_2R_2	3
cDe/cde	R_0r	1

D^u is significant, because if undetected in a donor it can stimulate anti-D in a dd patient. D^u subjects, transfused D Positive blood, can make anti-D, although this is a rare occurrence. D^u is more common in the Negro population.

Allelic antigens. Alleles at the Cc locus include C^w (1 per cent of UK population), C^x and C^u (comparable to D^u). Alleles at the Ee locus include E^w, E^u (comparable to D^u) and e^s (typically in blood from negro persons).

Compound antigens. Compound antigens occur in the Rhesus system as a product of two genes linked on a chromosome. These are defined by antibodies reacting only with the compound antigen, and not with the antigens on their own. These compound antigens are ce or f, Ce, cE CE and ce^s or V. G is not a compound antigen. It is present in all gene complexes except *cde* and *cdE*.

Missing Rh antigens. -D-/-D-: Cells of this group give negative reactions with antisera to C, c, C^w, E and e. The red cells possess more D antigen than normal, and can be completely agglutinated by some incomplete anti-D sera. C^wD- and cD- have also been described. Rh_{null}: These cells show no reactions with any Rhesus antisera. This appears to be due to a block in production of the required precursor to the Rhesus antigens.

Antibodies of the Rhesus system. Naturally-occurring antibodies within the Rhesus system are rare. Occasional examples, mainly anti-E, have been described. Rhesus antibodies are usually the result of sensitisation by pregnancy, transfusion, or injection of blood or blood products.

I blood group system

Antigens. The red cells of a normal adult carry the antigen I and a small amount of antigen i. Cord blood red cells however, carry antigen i and only react weakly with anti-I. Between birth and eighteen months of age the i antigen of the infant is gradually replaced by I. I antigen strength shows considerable variation in normal individuals. In addition the expected Ii antigen strengths are altered in diseases such as hypoplasia, acute leukaemia and megaloblastic anaemia.

The very rare adults who group as i have only a trace of I antigen on their cells. They are divided into i_1 and i_2.

Antibodies. Anti-I is present as an autoantibody in the serum of many adults as a cold agglutinin. It is usually a harmless antibody which does not cause cell destruction because of its low titre and low thermal amplitude.

In haemolytic anaemia of the 'cold' type the typical antibody is also anti-I. This is an IgM antibody present in high titre, active at a relatively high temperature (30°C) as a potent cold agglutinin and binds complement. It may also be associated with mycoplasma pneumonia.

Anti-i is unusual. It may occur in the serum of patients with reticulosis and with glandular fever.

P blood group system

Antigens. 74 per cent of Caucasians carry the antigens PP_1 and are called group P_1. There is a marked variation in antigen strength. The remaining 26 per cent carry the antigen P alone and are called P_2. Rare individuals have no detectable antigen and are called p. A further extremely rare antigen P^k is found mainly in Finland.

Antibodies. Anti-P_1. This antibody is frequently found in the serum of P_2 people, as a naturally-occurring IgM antibody causing agglutination in the cold. Occasional examples are active at higher temperatures. Strong anti-P_1 has been found in the serum of P_2 patients with hydatid cysts and anti-P_1 can be neutralized by hydatid cyst fluid.

Anti-*P*. This antibody has been found in the serum of all the rare P^k subjects. It will react with P_1 and P_2 cells.

Donath-Landsteiner antibody. The antibody present in the serum of patients with paroxysmal cold haemoglobinuria has an anti-P specificity. This antibody is an IgG and sensitises cells only at a low temperature but haemolysis occurs at 37°C.

Anti-P+P_1 +P^k (formerly called anti-Tj^a) is a powerful haemolytic antibody present in all p subjects.

MNSs blood group system

Antigens. The MNSs system is a complex system containing more than 30 antigens. The genes controlling M and N are closely linked to the genes controlling Ss and are inherited as a linked pair. s is more commonly complexed with N and S with M. The phenotypes and frequency are shown in Table 8.5.

Rare alleles of MN include N_2, M^g, M^c, M_1 and M^v. Further antigens associated with the MNSs system include Mi^a, Hu, He, Vr, Ny^a, Mt^a, St^a, Ri^a, Cl^a and Sul.

Antibodies. These are Anti-M and anti-N. Each is unusual in human sera, the rare examples presenting as cold agglutinins. Cases of haemolytic disease of the newborn due to anti-M have been described. Where an anti-M is active above 30°C it may cause a transfusion reaction. Anti-S is more commonly an immune IgG antibody and may cause transfusion reactions and haemolytic disease of the newborn.

Table 8.5 MNS system

Phenotype	% incidence in Caucasians
MNSs	24
MNs	22
Ns	15
MSs	14
Ms	8
MS	6
NSs	6
MNS	4
NS	1

Anti-s is very rare but has been the cause of haemolytic disease of the newborn.

Anti-U was origianlly thought to be anti-Ss but is now considered as a separate antibody occurring only in Negroes of the S^u group.

Lutheran blood group system

Antigens. The well defined antigens are Lu^a and Lu^b (Table 8.6).

Table 8.6 Lutheran system

Phenotype	% incidence in Caucasians
$Lu^{(a-b+)}$	92·3
$Lu^{(a+b+)}$	7·5
$Lu^{(a+b-)}$	0·2

Further linked antigens include Lu 4, Lu 5, Lu 6, Lu 7 and Lu 8 having a high incidence, and Lu 9 which is a low-incidence antigen.

Antibodies. Anti-Lu^a is an uncommon antibody, which may be naturally occurring or immune. It is most frequently a saline agglutinin with an optimum activity between 12 and 18°C.

Anti-Lu^b is also rare but reacts with 99·8 per cent of all blood samples and hence makes it difficult to find compatible blood. It will react as a saline agglutinin at room temperature or may be detected by an indirect antiglobulin technique.

Kell blood group system

Antigens. The Kell system also involves three linked alleles K:k, Kp^a:Kp^b, Js^a:Js^b (Table 8.7).

Table 8.7 Kell system

Phenotype	% incidence Caucasian	Negroid
KK	0·2	0·0?
Kk	8·8	3·5
kk	91·0	96·5
Kp$^{(a+b-)}$	0·0?	0·0?
Kp$^{(a+b+)}$	2·0	0·0?
Kp$^{(a-b+)}$	98·0	99·9
Js$^{(a+b-)}$	0·0?	1·1
Js$^{(a+b+)}$	0·0?	18·4
Js$^{(a-b+)}$	99·99	80·5

Further linked antigens are Ul^a K_{11} K_{12} K_{13} and Ku and KL. Ko red cells lack all the antigens of the Kell complex. The Kx antigen has been described on erythrocytes, leucocytes and platelets. It is utilised in the production of Kell antigens. Absence of Kx in erythrocytes gives the abnormal group McLeod which shows a weak reaction with antibodies of the Kell system. Absence of Kx on neutrophil leucocytes is associated with a defect of transport across the cell membrane and a lack in bactericidal activity. Some boys with X-linked chronic granulomatous disease have the McLeod phenotype, and lack Kx.

Antibodies. Anti-K is seldom naturally occurring. It is best detected by the indirect antiglobulin technique.

Anti-k is rare, due to the low incidence of KK individuals. When present, it is an immune antibody, and causes difficulty in finding compatible blood.

Anti-Kp^a, -Kp^b, -Js^a and -Js^b are rare.

Duffy blood group system

Antigens. The allelic genes Fy^a, Fy^b and Fy give rise to 4 phenotypes. These show a marked variation between the Negroid and Caucasian populations (Table 8.8).

Antibodies. Anti-Fy^a is most frequently an immune IgG antibody. Since the Fy^a antigen is destroyed by proteolytic enzymes, an indirect antiglobulin technique is required using complement-rich serum.

Anti-Fy^b antigen is destroyed by proteolytic enzymes, an indirect antiglobulin technique is required using complement-rich serum.

Anti-Fy^b is rare; it requires the indirect antiglobulin test for its detection.

Table 8.8   Duffy system

Phenotype	% incidence Caucasian	Negroid
$Fy^{(a+b-)}$	17	9
$Fy^{(a+b+)}$	49	1
$Fy^{(a-b+)}$	34	22
$Fy^{(a-b-)}$		68

Kidd blood group system

Antigens. The Kidd antigens are Jk^a and Jk^b (Table 8.9).

The group $Jk^{(a-b-)}$ has not been found in Caucasians or Negroes, but has been described in Hawaii.

Antibodies. Both anti-Jk^a and -Jk^b are infrequent. When present they are usually immune IgG antibodies and active by the indirect anti-globulin technique.

Table 8.9   Kidd system

Phenotype	% incidence English population
$Jk^{(a+b-)}$	25
$Jk^{(a+b+)}$	50
$Jk^{(a-b+)}$	25

Xg blood groups

The Xg^a antigen is the product of a gene on the X chromosome. Using an anti-Xg^a serum individuals may be grouped as Xg^a+ and Xg^a-.

Leucocyte and platelet antigens

Both leucocytes and platelets not only have many of the red-cell antigens but additional ones common to all tissues in the body.

Antigens also present on erythrocytes

The ABH antigens are present on leucocytes and platelets, but in a much weaker form. Ii antigens are present as in red cells and show the same adult/infant variation as in red cells. M, N and P antigens have been described. Rhesus antigens have not been detected.

Antigens specific for leucocytes and platelets

Specific leucocyte systems include the 5 system containing the antigens 5a and 5b, and also the NAᵢ system.

The P1^A system (previously called Zw) occurs only in platelets, 97 per cent of samples being P1^{A1}-positive. The Ko system of platelets contains the antigens Ko^a and Ko^b. A P1^E antigen has also been identified.

Antigens of the HLA system. These antigens occur on leucocytes, platelets, reticulocytes and most tissue cells, but not on mature red cells. They are important in matching donor and recipient in transplantation of organs such as the kidney. Four principal HLA-loci have been identified in man on chromosome 6. Each child has one such chromosome from each parent. Several possible alleles may occupy each locus. However, the chance of an identical HLA sibling being found is one in four. HLA-typing is carried out by incubating the patients lymphocytes against known sera (obtained from transfused patients and multigravidae) in the presence of complement. A reaction is indicated by cell death and hence uptake of the dye trypan blue which is excluded by viable cells.

Serum protein antigen systems

Due to antigenic differences in plasma proteins, multiple transfusions may also result in the formation of antibodies to protein antigens, particularly immunoglobulin antigenic determinants. There are two systems in which the antigens are well defined, namely Gm and Inv.

Gm System. The antigens are carried on the gamma chains of IgG. There are at least 25 Gm antigens which have been numbered. These are inherited as codominants at a single complex locus. Different Gm antigens are associated with different IgG subclasses, and most are located on the Fc piece of the molecule.

Km System. Km specificities occur on kappa chains and therefore occur in all immunoglobulin classes. There are three Km factors, 1, 2 and 3.

Antibodies to IgM and IgA determinants have also been recorded. Antibodies to plasma protein antigens may be the cause of febrile transfusion reactions, and necessitate the transfusion of washed red cells.

Part 2

The haematology department

9

The haematology department—organisation and management

The haematological team have two important roles, *viz.*, the clinical care of patients with blood disorders on the one hand, and the provision of a service for haematological investigation on the other.

The role of the clinical haematologist in the care of patients is no different from that of any other physician concerned with patient care. The development of a haematology department into a centre of excellence depends, among other factors, upon a high level of clinical competence as well as upon a high level of laboratory investigation. Increasingly the latter requires the provision of sophisticated and expensive equipment.

Laboratory design. In a hospital of 500–1000 beds the haematology department is conveniently divided into a number of sub-sections: (1) A laboratory mainly concerned with cell-counting procedures, preparation of blood films, sedimentation rates, etc.; (2) Blood Transfusion serology and other aspects of haematological immunolgy; (3) Coagulation; (4) B_{12} and folate assays and possibly related procedures; (5) 'Special' tests such as haemoglobin variants, haemolytic anaemia studies as well as developmental work; (6) Radioisotopes; (7) A record section, which in a large hospital will probably be computerized, and (8) Specimen Reception. These sections should be accommodated in separate rooms or laboratories within the haematology complex.

Working practice in haematology has changed considerably over the past few years and will continue to change with the continued introduction of more sophisticated apparatus. Benches should be easily moveable to provide ready access to all sides of bulky apparatus for maintenance and servicing. Large bench-type trolleys allow easy access to apparatus whilst permitting experimentation with positioning to allow work-flow modification. Bench tops should be constructed of impervious materials to permit easy disinfection and

Table 9.1 The haematology laboratory

Section	Suggested staffing level	Investigations undertaken
Routine blood counting	Senior Chief MLSO* / 1 Chief MLSO / 2 Senior MLSO / 5 MLSO / 3 Junior MLSO	Blood counts, E.S.R., platelet counts, reticulocytes counts, routine and special staining.
Blood Transfusion and Immunology	1 Chief MLSO / 1 Senior MLSO / 2 MLSO / 2 Junior MLSO	Blood grouping and compatability testing, antenatal testing, antigen and antibody identification. Perhaps tissue antibody and immunoglobulin work.
Coagulation	1 Senior MLSO / 1 Junior MLSO	The investigation of hypo- and hypercoagulable states and anticoagulant control.
Microbiological assay Radioisotopes	1 Senior MLSO / 1 Junior MLSO / ½ Chief or Senior MLSO	B_{12} and folate assay, figlu and methylmalonate tests. ^{51}Cr, ^{59}Fe, ^{57}Co(^{58}Co), ^{3}H, ^{125}I, ^{32}P, studies including surface counting.
'Special' investigations	1 Senior MLSO / 2 MLSO or Junior MLSO	Haemoglobin studies, haemolytic anaemia studies, ferritin, deoxyuridine suppression.
Specimen Reception	3–4 Clerks, preferably trained to operate computer terminals.	

*MLSO = Medical Laboratory Scientific Officer.

washing down to take place. Floors should be covered with non-slip surfacing. All rooms should be provided with adequate hand-washing facilities and there should be rest-rooms and cloakroom facilities within the complex for the use of all staff.

Modern blood counting machines produce large quantities of potentially hazardous waste and these should be plumbed into the drainage system directly in order to avoid sink contamination and leak hazards.

Noise is often an ill-considered hazard and noisy machinery, particularly computer terminals, should be well sound proofed. Air conditioning is often necessary where laboratories house large pieces of apparatus, particularly refrigerators, which discharge significant amounts of heat into the laboratory.

There is no longer the same need for extensive washing-up facilities in modern haematology laboratories since much of the small apparatus now used is disposable but sterilizing facilities should be available so that potentially contaminated waste may be safely disposed of. The use of bulky packaged reagents make it necessary to have adequate storage rooms and there should be a flammable goods store away from the main laboratory for the storage of stains and solvents.

A separate quiet microscopy room should be provided; a delicate instrument room with sturdy concrete benches for balances and spectrophotometers and a horizontal laminar flow cabinet (outflow) to protect work from contamination when materials are being prepared for patient injection.

Blood Transfusion laboratories should permit staff to work free from interruption by telephone and visitors. A trained reception clerk should deal with routine telephone calls, visitors and samples.

Blood sample collection. The haematology laboratory in a 1000-bed hospital may expect to receive between 300–500 blood count specimens per day. Out-patient samples and urgent samples will arrive throughout the working day but for the bulk of non-urgent ward samples the timing of specimen collection is critical to the efficient organisation of the laboratory. If the majority of non-urgent samples are available early in the day it will often be possible to return reports to the wards by the end of that day.

Venous blood samples are required for most laboratory tests and these should be collected by a team of phlebotomists trained and managed by the laboratory. This will also ensure that relatively few unsuitable samples will be received. Phlebotomy is particularly suitable for part-time workers since the bulk of specimen collection will be early in the working day.

Laboratory records. More and more laboratories are turning to computers to cope with the mass of data when large numbers of samples enter the laboratory.

Computers may be used (1) to compile work-sheets, (2) to store test results on patients' files, (3) to draw attention to work outstanding so that ordered tests are not overlooked, (4) to provide quality control data, (5) to compile work statistics so that costing may be carried out and changes in work patterns brought to light, and (6) to print final reports either singly or, perhaps more usefully, cumulative reports so that clinicians may compare current and previous data.

Computer systems may be on-line or off-line. Off-line systems have the considerable disadvantage that laboratory data has to be prepared for computer entry by the use of remote, tape-producing terminals. There are inevitably delays in this kind of system and frequent errors which are only noticed when attempts are made to feed data to the computer. On-line systems are more expensive but considerably more convenient.

A typical on-line system might consist of a hospital computer with a number of users including all the laboratories and all should have access to a master file of patient identities maintained by the hospital records department. Haematology would have a number of work stations on-line: (1) Reception—where requests would be entered with patient identity, location, consultant, etc.; (2) a Blood Count Terminal with a counting machine on-line so that counts would be entered directly onto the patient file. Facilities on this terminal might include an identity check against the work file, indications of changes in key parameters since the last test, counter errors in calculated parameters (MCH, PCV, MCHC) and on-going quality control both on standard samples and in the form of populations means; (3) a differential WBC terminal with electronic tally counters on-line; (4) a 'signing-out' terminal where comments on the appearance of the blood film or the assessment of the data may be entered; (5) a number of visual-display units with access to cumulative haematology records, hospital master index, work sheet display, and a results edit facility; (6) entry terminals for other tests. A particularly useful facility is one which allows the patients' blood group to be entered onto his master index record by blood transfusion staff; this will give instant access to patients' blood groups.

A crucial feature of any pathology computer system is the method of entering patient identity. Pathology work sheets must be capable of rapid generation and this effectively rules out full keyboard entry of data. A rapid and convenient data entry procedure is the use of bar codes readable by means of light-sensitive pens. Patients' hospital numbers may be entered into the system by this means and by the use of bar-code dictionaries location, consultant and tests requested may be entered.

Blood transfusion records. Proper records are mandatory in blood transfusion work. They should be designed not only to avoid clerical errors but also to ensure that the chances of mishap are minimal. Separate day books on preprinted sheets should be used to record details of grouping results, cross-matching procedures and antenatal work. These day books should record full patient identity as well as the actual working results of serological tests which are written directly into this book. The cross-matching book has a record of the full patient identity and location, details about the units of blood being cross matched and finally the actual results of compatability tests.

Reports on blood groups should utilize the colour code used to designate different blood groups on units of blood (blue for group O, yellow for group A, pink for group B, white for group AB with black lettering on Rhesus positive blood and red lettering on Rhesus negative blood). These coloured labels should be attached to the form reporting the blood group. Thus ward and theatre staff will become accustomed to group O patients whose report has a blue label with group O on it receiving a unit of group O blood with a corresponding blue label etc. The form that accompanies the cross-matched unit of blood back to the ward or theatre should contain two columns for the signatures of two persons who have confirmed that the identity stated on the blood unit corresponds to the person receiving the blood. This form is retained in the patient's folder.

Quality control
This is the means by which results within the laboratory are kept within acceptable levels of accuracy and precision.

Haemoglobin. In 1964 the International Committee for Standardis-ation in Haematology adopted the cyanmethaemoglobin method as the standard method for the estimation of haemoglobin, and the World Health Organisation established an International Haemiglobin-cyanide Reference Preparation in 1968. The standard is prepared by diluting haemoglobin in Drabkin's solution and the haemoglobin content determined by its extenction at 540 nm. Commerical solutions of known haemoglobin values are available. A similar solution can be prepared in the laboratory, its haemoglobin content being determined by its extinction at 540 nm. The standards are stable up to one year. These methods have supplanted earlier methods by which haemo-globin content was determined by iron content or by oxygen-carrying capacity of the blood sample. This solution can be used as a primary standard against which a batch of specimens can be read, to calibrate secondary standards and to set automatic blood counters.

Cell counts. Standards for cell counts are more difficult to prepare. White blood cells have a very short life in fresh samples. Osmium-tetroxide, formalin, tannic acid and glutaraldehyde have all been used to fix red cells so that they have a longer laboratory life as a standard. Commercial firms have been more successful but their methods usually are not disclosed. Fixed avian or reptilian red cells have been used as white cell counting standards and these may be added to the red cell preparations. Particles of polystyrene, latex, pollen and yeast have all been tried. Standards for platelet counting equipment are available, but the nature of the material has not been disclosed.

Calibration of these fixed cell preparations poses another problem. Values can be assigned on the basis of measurement in carefully controlled automatic counters. Another way is to test the preparation in a number of laboratories and assign a mean value to these preparations. Such preparations should be used as primary standards and used to assign values to 'secondary standards'. These are blood samples available in relatively large volumes and stored in aliquots that can be tested periodically throughout the working day.

Coagulation. The reliability of individual tests in coagulation, such as prothrombin time, kaolin-cephalin time or calcium thrombin time, depend on the quality of the reagents used, the care exercized in the collection and processing of the patient's blood and on the suitability of the control (normal) plasma. Carefully calibrated reagents are available for many coagulation tests, particularly the prothrombin time (Ch. 22). Laboratories that handle up to 20 prothrombin times or partial thromboplastin times per day should always test patient's plasma and control plasma in parallel, to ensure that the test is working. Laboratories that carry out many more tests can, in addition, plot the daily mean values as such or by a cusum method in order to observe long term trends.

The problem of the quality control of coagulation factor assays are similar to those encountered in clinical chemistry. The concentration of the coagulation factor in the patient's plasma is expressed as a percentage of the concentration of the reference plasma. The reference plasma can be a pool of freshly collected normal plasma or a freeze-dried plasma. Freeze-dried reference plasmas are provided as part of national or international calibration schemes or are available commercially. The comparison of test to reference plasma is carried out by a parallel line assay, that is, an assay of several dilutions of both plasmas. The results can be either plotted and read off a graph, or calculated using a programmable calculator. Laboratories that perform many such assays find it necessary to include two different reference plasmas in each run in order to calculate their ratio and in this way confirm the validity of the assay. Weekly results are plotted on a cusum chart or as an overall mean for the week or day. Many coagulation factors are labile on storage and reference plasma have a short shelf life; for this reason careful follow up of trends on the quality control charts is essential.

Blood transfusion standards. In blood transfusion serology quality control is achieved through controls of antisera, standard cells and standard reagents.

The antisera must be specific for the antigen against which they are directed and should detect that antigen in homozygous or heterozygous form. At the same time antisera must not react with cells lacking the antigen. Thus they must not have contaminating iso- or autoagglutinins, cold agglutinins; nor must they have any tendency to rouleaux formation. In every batch of tests therefore, a positive control is included of cells containing a single dose of the antigen in its weakest available form, and a negative control using cells lacking the antigen, but containing antigen to the most usual contaminating antibody. Examples are shown below.

Antiserum	Positive Cells	Negative Cells
Anti A	A_2 or A_2B	O and B
Anti D	O R_1r	ABrr

Reagent cells used for antibody detection are used fresh, at their optimum antigen strength. Their antigen content and agglutinability are controlled with every test using antisera of known specificity and strength.

Certain techniques are particularly vulnerable to fluctuation in quality. Undermodification in an enzyme technique gives falsely weak or negative results; overmodification gives false positives. Sensitivity of enzyme-treated cells is therefore controlled by a selected weak antibody. Antiglobulin tests are made invalid by minute globulin contamination. Cells weakly coated with globulin are used to control both the technique and the results obtained.

New batches of reagents such as albumin, enzyme and antiglobulin, are tested for sensitivity using serial dilutions of an antibody of known strength, in comparison with existing reagents.

Reproducibility of serial results as in antibody titration or quantitation can be checked against an International anti-D standard or a local standard may be checked against this, and then used in parallel with each batch of antibody measurements.

Statistical analysis of numerical results. Statistical methods are used in quality control where the result is a numerical value. The output of results from automatic blood counting machines may be analyzed. Means and standard deviation are calculated and, by the use of truncation limits (that is, results outside certain limits being excluded) mean values will remain remarkably constant from day to day. Acceptable limits of variation of mean values are determined and adjustments may be made when results stray outside of these limits. Computers may provide a running mean throughout the working day and thus errors in calibration may be more easily detected.

Cumulative sum or cusum methods may be used to detect drift away from correct calibration values. The basic calculation in their preparation involves subtracting a known or reference value from each value or mean value for an estimation, and accumulating the difference between each result and the constant value. Thus a haemoglobin value should be 13·8 g and if a series of values over eight days read 13·9, 13·9, 13·8, 14·0, 14·0, 13·9, 14·1, 14·1, the difference from the 'true' value to be added are +0·1, +0·1, 0, +0·2, +0·2, 01, 0·3 and +0·3. The cusum reads 0·1, 0·2, 0·2, 0·4, 0·6, 0·7, 1·0, 1·3. The drift from the true value is thus accentuated. It is essential to assign the true value accurately and this makes cusum plots more useful for single standards than for mean values where there may be great difficulty in assigning an accurate value or 'best mean'.

Where cumulative records are available earlier tests on a patient may serve as a very important control for current tests. A low MCV and MCH may mean iron-deficiency or thalassaemia or anaemia of chronic disorders, but normal values in earlier counts exclude thalassaemia and indicate an acquired disorder.

Controls in automatic blood counters. The Coulter Counter Model S is widely used and though these comments refer to this machine they are applicable to equipment from other manufacturers. Initially the machine must be set to produce 'correct' values with a blood sample. Thereafter, other blood samples will be read in relation to the initial setting. In practice the haemoglobin value of the blood sample used in setting up the machine is determined with a cyanmethaemoglobin standard and the red and white cell counts are determined with a cell counter of the Coulter Counter Model F type. The PCV is determined by the microhaematocrit method. The machine is set so that the correct values are obtained with this particular blood sample. Some will prefer to make this initial setting with a commercial standard blood. Further a choice has to be made as to whether the PCV will match the microhaematocrit value which on average is 1·4 per cent higher than the true PCV because of trapped plasma or whether the setting will be that of a true PCV. In the latter case the machine PCV taking the average for ten blood samples is 1·4 per cent less than the average haematocrit PCV for these same samples.

Once the machine has been set it is necessary to ensure that the calibration remains within acceptable limits. One method of doing this is to calculate the means of all samples tested throughout the day or the mean values of samples after 'abnormal' samples have been excluded. Thus only blood samples with haemoglobin values between 12 to 17 g/100 ml may be used. These mean values are plotted on a chart and drift outside accepted ranges may indicate the need to re-calibrate the machine. Larger errors in machine calibration are detected by testing standard blood samples at the beginning and regularly throughout the working day. These standards may be bloods tested the previous day or large volumes of blood which have been standardized previously. With a computer an on-going mean may be available on a display screen. An alternative method of plotting the mean values is by the cusum method described earlier.

Other aspects. Controls for assay of vitamin B_{12} and folate, abnormal haemoglobins, red cells enzyme determinations etc., are more difficult to obtain. In microbiological assay sera from patients with low values are stored and aliquot included in each batch. Known amounts of pure vitamin B_{12} or folate are added to specimens and recoveries noted. Mean values for assay batches are plotted and batches outside predetermined limits are discarded. With folate assays haemolysates in aqueous ascorbate stored frozen provide the most satisfactory assay standards. All too often the failure of a result to correlate with the clinical state may be the clue to a poorly functioning assay.

Maintenance of haemoglobin solutions representing different abnormalities represent the usual way abnormal haemoglobins are monitored.

In addition to the quality control procedures described, most countries have a central organisation which distributes test samples to laboratories for examination. The true value is taken to be the mean result obtained by pooling the results from all the participating laboratories or the mean result obtained by a group of selected laboratories. This is a guide to the laboratories performance and in some countries a consistently poor performance has led to the laboratory being closed down.

Other aspects of laboratory organisation

Slide storage. Maintenance of blood count data on individual patients should go hand in hand with storage of the corresponding blood films. This makes it possible to review a haematological problem. Similarly marrow films should be retained. With modern slide storage cabinets large numbers of slides covering several years can be kept in a relatively small space. Slides of special interest can be filed in relation to diagnosis so that trays of slides of patients with different diseases are available for teaching purposes.

Provision of 24 hour service. Staff have an obligation to provide laboratory services after normal working hours. This duty should be spread as widely as possible among staff so that individuals should not be required to be on call more frequently than one in 8–10 nights or week-ends. The number of investigations offered out of hours should be limited to those tests that may be required to reach a decision for urgent management only. In haematology, these are blood count, inspection of a stained blood film, platelet count, coagulation screen, sickle cell test, blood grouping and cross matching of blood and direct antiglobulin test.

Staff morale. Since the major role of the haematology department is the carrying out of large numbers of often indistinguishable blood counts the risk of boredom and poor staff performance is high. Good working conditions, regular rotation of staff through different sections of the laboratory, teaching and discussion sessions during working hours and delegation of authority to those working in different sections of the laboratory are all useful.

Part 3

Blood diseases

10

Signs and symptoms in blood diseases

Primary disorders of the blood are far less common than changes in the blood secondary to disease elsewhere.

Anaemia

Symptoms. The effects of anaemia on the patient are the result of reduction in the oxygen-carrying capacity of the blood. The severity of the symptoms relate to the level of haemoglobin and to the length of time over which the anaemia developed.

The patient feels tired and weak. He or she is short of breath on exertion particularly on climbing stairs and is aware of the heart beating (palpitations). In severe anaemia or in an older patient with narrowed blood vessels in the heart, there may be chest pain related to exercise and disappearing on rest (anginal pain) due to insufficient oxygen reaching the heart muscle.

Swelling of the feet particularly at the end of the day may be due to mild heart failure precipitated by the anaemia. There may be pain in the legs on exertion again relieved on rest (intermittent claudication) due to diminished oxygen supply to the limbs.

There may be loss of appetite, sometimes difficulty with swallowing (dysphagia) and a feeling of a lump in the throat. The latter symptom often occurs in severe iron-deficiency anaemia. Mouth and tongue may be sore particularly after hot drinks. These symptoms are due to failure to replace cells lining the mouth and tongue in iron, vitamin B_{12} or folate deficiency.

There may be a tingling or a pins and needles sensation in the hands and feet. Nails may be unusually brittle.

Compensatory mechanisms. In order to make maximum use of the remaining haemoglobin, the blood is circulated more rapidly round the body. This is brought about by the heart pumping the blood around more rapidly, that is, there is an increased cardiac output. This 'high output state' is accompanied by an opening up of small vessels in the tissues so that there is less resistance to the movement of blood and the hands tend to feel warm. In time this extra stress on the heart coupled with reduced oxygen supply can lead to heart failure. Chronic reduction of oxygen to the heart in older people can lead to damage to the muscle (seen as an accumulation of fat in muscle fibres) and if the amount of fluid in the circulation is suddenly increased by blood transfusion, the heart can fail.

The total blood volume is always maintained. Thus as the amount of red cells falls the plasma increases. With a very slow onset of anaemia the patient slowly adjusts to the new circumstances and may complain of few symptoms until the anaemia is severe.

With increasing anaemia the oxygen comes off the red cells more readily due to an increase in the level of 2,3-diphosphoglycerate which shifts the oxygen dissociation curve to the right.

Signs. The anaemic patient is pale. Not only is this evident in skin, but also in the nails, tongue and conjunctivae. He or she may be breathless and veins in the neck may be prominent.

If there is a shortening of red cell life span the plasma bilirubin level may be elevated. This may give rise to jaundiced sclera. When slight jaundice is combined with severe anaemia as in pernicious anaemia the patient's skin acquires a characteristic lemon-yellow colour. White hair and blue eyes complete the text book picture of untreated pernicious anaemia.

The tongue may be smooth and shiny and there may be cracks at the angles of the mouth (angular stomatitis). The nails in severe iron deficiency may be spoon shaped (koilonychia) instead of being normally curved. Feet may be swollen and the examination of the heart in addition to the two normal heart sounds may show an additional soft blowing systolic murmer—a haemic murmer. Not uncommonly the temperature may be elevated in untreated pernicious anaemia.

Platelet lack

When the platelet count is unduly low the patient may notice that he or she bruises after very minor bumps or even apparently spontaneously. This may be on any part of the body. A more characteristic feature of lack of platelets is the appearance of small red spots due to rupture of capillaries. Purpura tends to be frequent on dependent parts such as the legs and most noticeable in the arm after a tourniquet or blood pressure cuff has been applied. On occasion the first evidence of something untoward may be a prolonged nose bleed. Blood in the urine (haematuria) may occur. In addition to these manifestations haemorrhagic areas may be seen inside the eye when the retina is inspected through an ophthalmoscope and inside the mouth.

Coagulation disorder

These are bleeding disorders due to defects in one or other coagulation factor in plasma. Though rare they may be congenital and hence a family history of a similar disorder is important. Bleeding into tissues (as opposed to bleeding into skin in platelet disorders) is the feature. Bleeding may be into a large joint (knee, ankle, elbow), into muscle such as thigh, buttock, arm and may occur in response to minor trauma. Once a bleed occurs it is extremely painful and may progress and persist for many days.

Prolonged bleeding from wounds and lacerations is another feature but punctate bleeding as in platelet defects, does not occur. The commonest condition here is haemophilia.

Neutrophil lack

Lack of neutrophils or neutrophils that do not function in a normal manner, render the patient unusually susceptible to infection. In young children this may manifest itself as repeated infections of the ears, nose and throat and by chest infections. If severe, the condition is fatal.

Acquired loss of neutrophils in adults most often result in a persistent and severe sore throat. Such a symptom in a patient taking a drug that is known on occasion to depress white cells, should alert one to the possibility of agranulocytosis. Other manifestations are the appearance of local infections at the site of minor skin trauma such as venepuncture sites, and a raised temperature. The most severe complication is septicaemia, a proliferation of bacteria in the blood stream. The patient has a rapid rise in temperature, shivering, muscle pains and shows signs of collapse.

A common symptom in chronic (but less severe) neutropenia is the appearance of frequent small shallow clean mouth ulcers that may be painful. These heal after a few days.

11

Disorders of white blood cells

Morphological abnormalities;   Leucocytosis
Leucopenia   Non-functioning neutrophils
Glandular fever

Morphological variations

Pelger-Huët anomaly. The neutrophil nucleus has either two lobes
or is a band form. (Fig. 11.1). It is inherited as a dominant
characteristic and the cells function quite normally. In megaloblastic
anaemia in such a patient more 'normal looking' neutrophils with three
or four lobes appear and these revert to the usual form after treatment.

Pelger-Huet
neutrophils

Fig. 11.1 A neutrophil polymorph with the Pelger-Huët anomaly.

Hereditary hypersegmentation of neutrophils. This too, is transmitted
as a dominant character, neutrophils having four or more nuclear
lobes. (Fig. 11.2).

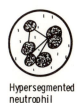

Hypersegmented
neutrophil

Fig. 11.2 A neutrophil polymorph with increased numbers of nuclear segments.

May-Hegglin anomaly. The cytoplasm of the neutrophil contains
round or oval, blue or grey-staining bodies termed *Döhle bodies*. (Fig.
11.3). It may be associated with a low platelet count, low white cell
count and occasional giant platelets. It is inherited in a dominant
manner.

Alder-Reilly anomaly. The neutrophil granules stain a deep purple colour due to excess mucopolysaccharide. It is transmitted as a recessive characteristic.

Chediak-Higashi syndrome. The cytoplasm of some neutrophils, lymphocytes and monocytes contain large purple staining granules. In neutrophils these replace the normal granules but this may appear as a solitary mass in lymphocytes and monocytes (Fig. 11.4). These structures are giant lysosomes. It is associated with failure of skin and eye pigmentation (albinism). It is inherited as a recessive and is usually fatal due to anaemia, low white and platelet counts.

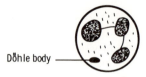

Döhle body

Fig. 11.3 Cytoplasmic (Döhle) bodies in the neutrophil polymorph in the May-Hegglin anomaly.

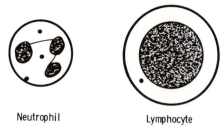

Neutrophil   Lymphocyte

in Chediak-Higashi Syndrome

Fig. 11.4 Abnormal cytoplasmic granules in Chediak-Higashi syndrome.

Neutral-lipid storage disease (Jordan's anomaly). Large lipid globules accumulate in all cells (Fig. 11.5). In blood films they appear as large vacuoles but take fat stains such as oil-R-O. They are most obvious in neutrophils. It is associated with a scaly skin disorder

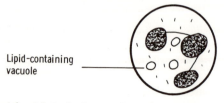

Lipid-containing vacuole

Fig. 11.5 Neutral-fat globules in the cytoplasm of neutrophil polymorphs in neutral-lipid storage disease.

(ichthyosis) and/or muscular wasting (dystrophy). It is part of a general disorder of fat metabolism

Toxic granulation. This describes the appearance of unusually prominent neutrophil granules associated with severe infections. It is often part of a leucocytosis but in early infection neutrophil numbers may be normal or even reduced.

Shift to the left. The normal distribution of nuclear lobes in neutrophils is as follows—unsegmented (4 per cent), two lobes (26 per cent) three lobes (48 per cent), four lobes (19 per cent) and five lobes (3 percent). In infection there is an increase in unsegmented and two lobed forms. This is called a shift to the left. Metamyelocytes, myelocytes and Döhle bodies may be present.

Shift to the right. Here there is an increase in four- and five-lobed forms and even six-lobed forms appear. This occurs chiefly in megaloblastic anaemia and less commonly in iron deficiency and renal failure (uraemia).

Anticoagulant changes. Many anticoagulants, particularly ethylene diamine tetra-acetic acid (EDTA, sequestrene) hasten degenerative change in white blood cells. The neutrophil lobes may become separated and stain as dense dark balls. Monocytes become vacuolated and the nucleus grossly lobulated. Lymphocytes are less affected but also develop nuclear lobulation. Changes start appearing after 2–3 hours of collection of the blood sample.

Nuclear sexing. A significant proportion of neutrophils in women have an appendage or drumstick which is due to the XX chromosome as opposed to XY in males (Fig. 11.6).

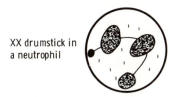

XX drumstick in a neutrophil

Fig. 11.6 Drumstick in the nucleus of the neutrophil polymorph in females.

Leucocytosis

Neutrophil leucocytosis. An increase in neutrophil numbers above $7500/\mu l$ occurs in infection due to many organisms including staphylococci, streptococci, gram-negative bacilli such as E. coli etc. Such infections may be local (abscess), chest infection (pneumonia), renal infection (pyelonephritis) etc. An increase in neutrophils also occurs in tissue injury such as burns, myocardial infarction, surgical operation etc. The increase in white cell count may be from 12000 to greater than $30000/\mu l$. It may be associated with toxic granulation and appearance of metamyelocytes and occasionally myelocytes in the blood. Earlier white cells do not appear. When the white cell count is very high, the term leukaemoid reaction has been used but blast cells are not present and this helps to distinguish the blood changes from those in leukaemia. Alkaline phosphatase can be quantitated in the neutrophils. It will be high in infection and low in leukaemia.

Eosinophilia is found in allergic diseases, parasitic infections, some skin diseases which may be allergic, and infrequently in other conditions like Hodgkin's Disease, polyarteritis nodosa etc.

Basophilia virtually only occurs in chronic myeloid leukaemia and myeloproliferative disorders.

Lymphocytosis. A permanent increase in lymphocytes in adults occurs only in chronic lymphocytic leukaemia. Young children tend to respond to a variety of infections with lymphocytosis when adults would respond with a rise in neutrophils. Very high counts may be seen in whooping cough (pertussis infection) and a virus disease called acute infectious lymphocytosis. Some increase may be seen in hepatitis, in glandular fever associated with EB virus, cytomegalic virus or toxoplasma infection.

Monocytosis is rare except in leukaemia.

Leucopenia
Clinically a low white cell count (less than 2000 neutrophils/μl) is as important as a high one but clinical symptoms do not appear until neutrophils are less than $500/\mu l$. Patients with neutropenia are at increased risk of infection which may be minor or overwhelming and rapidly fatal. Persistent neutropenia can be:

Secondary to other diseases. Some bacterial infections (typhoid, brucella), virus infections (influenza virus, or hepatitis virus), marrow infiltration (cancer or leukaemia) or removal of neutrophils by an avid spleen (hypersplenism, Felty's syndrome).

Due to therapy such as drugs (anti-thyroid, analgesics, anti-rheumatic, anti-mitotic, chloramphenicol). The list is vast. It can be due to radiotherapy.

Failure of production as in megaloblastic anaemia, aplastic anaemia, or for genetic reasons.

Autoimmune neutropenia. These tend to respond to steroid therapy.

Congenital neutropenias
These are found in early life and the more severely affected children die in the first 1-2 years of life from repeated infections. Milder cases

tend to improve particularly after puberty. A severe familial form transmitted in a recessive manner was described among the Lapps. These infants had repeated middle ear and chest infections.

In some patients the neutrophil count falls approximately every three weeks and remains very low for a few days (cyclical neutropenia). Preceding the blood changes the marrow empties of granulocytes, and thereafter recovers. At the time of the low count the patient may feel unwell and have a temperature. Antibiotic cover to coincide with the period of neutropenia may be required.

In chronic neutropenia the only complaint may be of repeated painful shallow mouth ulcers.

Impaired neutrophil function
Recurrent bacterial infections may be due to defective bactericidal activity of the polymorphonuclear leucocytes. This failure may be in defective neutrophil movement, in defective phagocytosis or in defective killing mechanisms within the neutrophils.

Defects of chemotaxis. Recurrent infections associated with impaired chemotaxis of neutrophils have been found in several infants. The defects may be absence of serum factors acting as opsonins the most significant being absence of complement (C_3, C_5) or there may be an intrinsic defect in the neutrophil so that they fail to migrate in the direction of chemotactic factors. Methods of assessment remain unsatisfactory and no one method will necessarily be abnormal in every case. These include skin windows, Boyden chambers and capillary tube assays.

Defects of phagocytosis. Delayed or absent phagocytosis when present, has been accompanied by other defects such as absence of opsonins. Phagocytosis is an energy-requiring process. Neutrophils have receptors for the Fc portion of IgG immunoglobulins and for certain components of complement and these link the neutrophil to the antibody-coated organism. Conditions where impairment of both phagocytosis and bacterial killing may occur include immunoglobulin deficiencies both congenital and acquired, abnormalities of the complement system, leukaemic leucocytes, and the effects of drugs and toxins including ethanol, cytotoxics and corticosteroids.

Defects of bacterial killing. These disorders include a number of intrinsic neutrophil defects leading to a failure of generation of hydrogen peroxide and superoxide radicles, possibly myeloperoxide deficiency and degranulation defects in the Chediak-Higashi syndrome. The commonest syndrome is chronic granulomatous disease presenting in the first year of life with suppurative lymphadenopathy, pneumonitis, dermatitis and enlarged liver and spleen. It may be inherited in either a sex-linked or autosomal manner. In these disorders organisms are phagocytosed normally but are not killed. Phagocytosis normally triggers off a burst of oxidative activity with production of superoxide anions and this fails to occur in these disorders. This pathway also leads to reduction of nitrobluetetrazolium (NBT) a test used in the diagnosis of this group of disorders.

Glandular fever (infectious mononucleosis)

This is a very common disease of young adults. It is frequent in general medical practice but patients only rarely need to come to hospital. The patient has fever, a sore throat, enlarged tender lymph glands and the spleen may be enlarged. The identical clinical and blood picture can be due to the Epstein-Barr (EB) virus, cytomegalic virus and toxoplasma gondii, but only infection with the EB virus result in heterophile (sheep-cell) antibodies in blood (positive Paul-Bunnell Test). Infection with the other agents give a Paul-Bunnell negative disease.

The virus can invade many tissues and hence the signs can be variable. Most patients have liver involvement—usually abnormal liver function tests but occasionally jaundice. The nervous system can be involved (headache, eye problems, paralyses). Skin rashes may appear.

The white cell count is usually raised and most of the rise is due to atypical lymphocytes. A usual count is 13 000 white cells of which 9000 are lymphocytes. The cells have a large fleshy monocyte-like nucleus and abundant rich royal blue cytoplasm. *Rarely* the neutrophil count may be reduced and platelet count may be low but usually they are normal. Haemoglobin is almost always normal unless there is associated iron deficiency. *Rarely* a haemolytic anaemia is present due to the production of an IgM immunoglobin of anti-i specificity.

The uncomplicated illness lasts 2–3 weeks and abnormal cells disappear from the blood in 1–3 months. There is no specific treatment.

The diagnostic test is the Paul-Bunnell. Human sera commonly have a factor that agglutinates sheep red blood cells. This factor has been called the 'heterophile antibody'. This antibody is removed by absorption of the serum with guinea-pig kidney. On the other hand the antibody in glandular fever is not affected by absorption with guinea-pig kidney and still agglutinates sheep cells after such treatment. This is a positive Paul-Bunnell Test. Generally a positive result with a dilution of serum of greater than 1 in 10 is significant.

The aetiological role postulated for the EB virus in glandular fever is based on the observation that individuals sero-negative against the EB virus become sero-positive after a typical attack of glandular fever. Further only sero-negative individuals are susceptible to an attack of glandular fever. However the virus can be recovered in only a minority of patients.

The infection often raises the titre of other antibodies and false positive results may occur in tests for syphilis and in the widal test for typhoid.

Reference

Cline M J, Golde D W 1977 Granulocytes and monocytes: function and functional disorders. In: Hoffbrand A V, Brain M C, Hirsh J (eds) Recent Advances in Haematology. Churchill Livingstone, Edinburgh, p 69–84

12

Disorders of red blood cells

Morphological abnormalities
Iron-deficiency anaemia
Megaloblastic anaemias

Morphological abnormalities

The terms listed below are used in describing the appearance of red blood cells in the stained blood film (Fig. 12.1).

Anisocytosis describes a greater variation in red cell size than is usual.

Poikilocytosis refers to the presence of pear-shaped red cells.

Polychromasia describes a retention of a grey coloration in some red cells with Romanowsky stains. This is indicative of RNA in such cells which are reticulocytes.

Macrocytosis indicates the presence of abnormally large red cells.

Microcytosis indicates the presence of abnormally small red cells. The terms, macrocytosis and microcytosis are also used for a high or low MCV respectively in the blood count.

Hypochromia which is associated with microcytosis, refers to pale staining red cells with thin rims of haemoglobin.

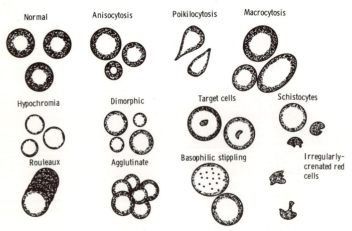

Fig. 12.1 Morphological abnormalities of red blood cells seen in stained blood films.

Dimorphic refers to the presence of two populations of red cells identified in a blood film, e.g. hypochromic and normochromic cells.

Target cells or leptocytes are thin flattened red cells the centre of which stain more densely.

Spherocytes are small densely staining round red cells which have lost their central concavity.

Elliptocytes or ovalocytes refer to a tendency for the red cells to be oval or elongated. It is an inherited trait.

Schistocytes refer to red cell fragments present in the stained film.

Rouleaux is the tendency for red cells to pack like piles of coins.

Agglutination is the tendency for red cells to clump together in groups often in thicker parts of the blood smear and where marked, may be due to a cold antibody.

Basophilic stippling or punctate basophilia refers to fine black stipples appearing in occasional stained red cells. It is abnormal if present in excess of 3 per 1000 red cells and occurs in lead poisoning, but also in megaloblastic anaemia etc. Such cells are polychromatic.

Howell-Jolly bodies are remains of normoblast nuclei appearing as small black round bodies in the red cell. It is found most often after the spleen has been removed or has undergone atrophy, but may be seen in severe dyshaemopoiesis such as megaloblastic anaemia.

Pappenheimer bodies are small dark staining spots in the red cell. These spots also show up when a Prussian-blue stain for iron is carried out, that is, they are iron-containing or siderotic granules and these red cells are siderocytes.

Irregularly-crenated red cells refer to distorted red cells seen after splenectomy, in drug-induced damage to red cells and sometimes in other disorders. It is contrasted with crenation commonly seen in films made from blood many hours after collection.

Acanthrocytes are spicules or spines in red cells seen in a rare condition of β-lipoproteinaemia wherein the lipid of the red cell gets eluted into the plasma. It is also seen in thyroid deficiency (hypothyroidism, myxoedema).

Iron-deficiency anaemia
Normal iron metabolism is discussed in Chapter 4.

Cause of iron deficiency
An overall lack of iron may arise if the loss of iron from the body is greater than the amount of iron absorbed from the diet. The principal causes are:

Increased iron loss, e.g. chronic bleeding;
Increased iron requirement, e.g. pregnancy, infancy;
Inadequate intake due to either a poor diet, or to impaired
intestinal absorption.

Blood loss. Most of the iron in the body is in the form of
haemoglobin in red blood cells. Bleeding is the most important way in
which iron is lost from the body and this takes place most often from
the intestinal tract in both sexes and by excessive menstrual bleeding
in women.

Bleeding in the gut may be from a *hiatus hernia* which is a protrusion
of part of the stomach through a gap in the diaphragm into the chest.
This may produce ulceration and some bleeding both as a result of
pressure by the diaphragm and from the passage of acid gastric juice
into the oesophagus which produces local damage. *Oesophageal varices*
are large veins which develop at the lower end of the oesophagus when
the liver is fibrosed (cirrhosis) and hence the normal venous blood flow
to the liver is blocked. These large veins bleed periodically. *Gastric* or
duodenal ulcers may erode blood vessels. Regular *salicylate* ingestion
(aspirin etc.) cause superficial gastric ulcers which bleed. A *cancer* of
the stomach, colon or rectum, *regional ileitis*, (an inflammatory disease
of small gut), *ulcerative colitis* (an inflammatory disease of large gut),
diverticulitis (pouches sticking out of the wall of the large gut which
may become inflamed) and *piles* are common causes of blood loss.
Capillary nodules (haemangiomata) in the gut wall may be very small
and be difficult to find even at operation, but can bleed profusely.
Hookworm infestation is a very important cause of blood loss since
worm infestation may be heavy and may result in daily loss of up to
250 ml of blood. In *hereditary haemorrhagic telangiectasia* there are
diffuse abnormal capillaries throughout the body. These may be seen
on the skin and in the mouth, nasopharynx and gut and any of these
may be the site of regular blood loss.

Excessive bleeding in menstruation (menorrhagia) is the most
important single cause of iron deficiency in women. Bleeding into the
urine is a less common cause of iron deficiency. *Blood donors*
particularly women giving blood regularly, often become iron
deficient.

Increased iron requirement. Pregnancy produces an increased need
for iron from a normal 1–2 mg per day to a maximum of 6 mg per day so
that the majority of women if not given oral iron, will become iron
deficient (Ch. 20).

Poor intake. Patients who suffer from excessive menstrual blood loss and women with anaemia in pregnancy often take a relatively *poor diet* which does not supply enough iron. Some 15 per cent of apparently healthy women have iron-deficiency anaemia.

Malabsorption of iron is important after operations on the stomach such as partial gastrectomy and occasionally in patients with glutensensitive enteropathy. The stomach normally converts a meal into a liquid state (chyme) which is passed on to the duodenum in a regular manner. After many gastric operations this function is lost so that unprepared food passes too rapidly past the upper gut where the iron is absorbed. Intestinal malabsorption should also be considered in some patients not responding to oral iron treatment, but failure to take their iron tablets is a more probable explanation.

Events in negative iron balance

Once there is negative iron balance, iron stores are used up. This is followed by a fall in the serum iron and thereafter a fall in haemoglobin level. Depletion of iron-containing enzymes develops last. (Fig. 12.2).

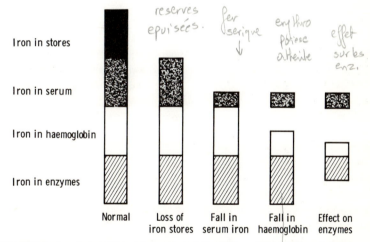

Fig. 12.2 In iron lack a fall in iron stores is followed by a fall in the serum iron level and thereafter a fall in haemoglobin level. Finally synthesis of iron-containing enzymes fails.

Clinical aspects

Patients complain of loss of energy, tiredness, shortness of breath, i.e. the signs and symptoms of anaemia described in chapter 10. A smooth sore tongue is common as is a characteristic irregularity (spooning) of the nails called koilonychia.

A combination of difficulty in swallowing, a band or mucosal web seen on X-ray after swallowing Barium at the back of the throat (pharynx) and iron-deficiency anaemia appears in the literature as the 'Plummer-Vinson' syndrome.

Diagnosis

There is anaemia and the MCV and MCH are low. Subsequently the MCHC falls. The more severe the anaemia the lower are these indices. The platelet count is often raised (400 000 to 500 000/μl) presumably as the response to chronic bleeding. The blood film shows hypochromic red cells. Some red cells may be elongated in the stained film (pencil cells). Occasionally hypersegmented neutrophils are prominent. The blood picture may be the same in two other conditions giving rise to small red cells—thalassaemia trait and anaemia of chronic disorders (particularly rheumatoid arthritis). Small red cells may be found in haemoglobinopathies and in hyperthroidism. Thalassaemia can often be suspected because the red cell count is relatively high. If the MCV is low, a red cell count above 5·5 million/μl favours thalassaemia, below 5·0 million favours iron-deficiency anaemia.

Iron deficiency can be confirmed by measuring the serum iron and iron-binding capacity. In iron deficiency the serum-iron level is low (below 60 μg/100 ml or 11 μmol/l) and iron-binding capacity raised (above 350 μg/100 ml or 63 μmol/l). In anaemia of chronic disorders *both measurements are low.* In uncomplicated thalassaemia trait both are normal. The serum ferritin is reduced generally below 10 ng per ml.

Another way of confirming a diagnosis of iron deficiency is by staining marrow aspirates for iron by Perls's method. The fatty fragment should be examined under lower power for dark green-staining, iron-containing cells. These will be absent in iron deficiency provided that a control marrow or section known to contain iron stained as a control, is positive.

The marrow in iron-deficiency anaemia, is generally of normal cellularity. The late erythroblasts have small, pyknotic, irregular and

Normoblast

Micronormoblast

Fig. 12.3 The micronormoblast showing irregular nucleus and ragged cytoplasm.

distorted nuclei and the cytoplasm is noticeably ragged. These cells are called micronormoblasts (Fig. 12.3).

Investigation
It is relatively easy to diagnose iron deficiency, more difficult and time-consuming to establish the cause.

Clinical history. Is the patient taking tablets or medicine (salicylates) that can cause bleeding? Does he or she come from a part of the world where hookworm is common? Does the patient have piles or notice blood when passing faeces? Is blood loss associated with menstrual periods unduly severe?

Gastro-intestinal blood loss. Biochemical tests on the faeces for occult blood loss are of great importance. The motion may look perfectly normal if there is no intestinal hurry despite containing several 100 ml of blood, because the blood has been altered by intestinal enzymes. Loss of as little as 6 ml blood daily is enough to lead to an iron-deficiency anaemia. Blood loss can be very intermittent, that is, none may be detected for many days when testing faeces for occult blood, and this can be followed by blood loss when the test becomes positive.

A quantitative way of measuring blood loss is to label the patients red blood cells with ^{51}Cr. The motions are collected and a venous blood sample collected with each batch of stools to serve as a standard. Both stools and blood are counted for radioactivity. Radioactivity in stools is readily translated into ml of blood lost per 24 hours. Similarly menstrual blood loss has been quantitated by collecting pads used into a container and measuring radioactivity.

Radiology. Barium meal and enema are important in detecting many lesions in the gastrointestinal tract already mentioned.

Sigmoidoscopy. An optical tube inserted into rectum and sigmoid colon enables the clinician to see bleeding lesions in the distal large gut.

Radioactive iron studies are of little help. Iron clearance from plasma is rapid and there is a very high utilization of the iron for haemoglobin formation. Iron absorption from the gut is augmented in iron deficiency (and normal pregnancy) but the maximum uptake is still only 4 mg iron per day.

The final proof in more complex cases may sometimes be sought in response to iron treatment given alone.

Management
Where possible the cause of the anaemia is identified and if amendable to treatment, is dealt with. This may include withdrawal of salicylate-containing medication. Surgery may be required in the case

of neoplasms and sometimes to search for an elusive cause of major gut haemorrhage such as a haemangioma.

Treatment for the anaemia consists of the administration inorganic iron tablets by mouth, 200 mg ferrous sulphate given three times daily being the most satisfactory. Intestinal upset is common on commencement of iron treatment and if troublesome is dealt with by a reduction in the dose of iron. Iron can also be given in relatively large amounts by injection (iron-dextran, iron-sorbitol). This should be used only under special circumstances where the patient cannot take or absorb iron by mouth. Iron is also given to prevent the development of iron deficiency in pregnancy where one tablet per day suffices.

Response to iron treatment
Response is less dramatic than treatment in megaloblastic anaemia. Except in severe anaemia reticulocytes only occasionally exceed 10 per cent in the second week and there is a steady rise in haemoglobin level at the rate of about 1·0 g per 100 ml each week. The rate of rise of the haemoglobin level is only marginally more rapid after parenteral injections of iron. Oral iron should be continued long enough to supply iron stores, that for four to six months.

Megaloblastic anaemias

The physiology of vitamin B_{12} and folic acid is discussed in Chapter 4. Anaemia due to lack of vitamin B_{12} or folate results in abnormally large red blood cells appearing in the blood (macrocytosis). The marrow shows changes which are called megaloblastic. By contrast, there are a number of disorders which also give rise to macrocytosis where the marrow generally remains normoblastic.

Normoblastic macrocytosis: Red cell hypoplasia and aplasia; myxoedema; sideroblastic anaemia; haemolytic anaemia; alcoholism; reticulocytosis.

Megaloblastic macrocytosis: Vitamin B_{12} deficiency; folic-acid deficiency; interference with DNA synthesis.

Recognition of a megaloblastic process
This is made by examination of the peripheral blood and, if necessary, the marrow.

Blood count. The earliest change in the blood count is a rise in the MCV while all else is still within normal limits. Thereafter the red cell count and haemoglobin concentration fall and when the red cell count is less than 2·0 million/μl the white cell count and platelet count fall. As the anaemia becomes more severe the MCV increases up to about

130–135 fl. The most severe cases have a red cell count of about 1 million/μl, WBC of 1000–2000/μl, and platelets of 20 000 to 50 000/μl.

Blood film. In the early stages there may be some difficulty in recognizing a minor degree of uniform macrocytosis in a blood film although the automatic blood counter records a raised MCV. As anisocytosis appears the oval macrocytes become more evident and red cell fragments and poikilocytes may be seen. The neutrophils show a shift to the right with an increase in the numbers of 5-and 6-lobed forms. If the patient has lost his or her spleen (atrophic as in coeliac disease and sickle-cell anaemia or removed surgically as part of a gastrectomy) postsplenectomy features appear in the stained blood film. These are Howell-Jolly bodies in the red cells, red cell fragments and red cell crenation, and there are more erythroblasts sometimes recognizably megaloblastic in character, than one expects.

Marrow. A fully developed peripheral blood picture is diagnostic of a megaloblastic process. In less anaemic patients the diagnosis should always be confirmed by marrow aspiration. The marrow shows megaloblastic haemopoiesis being recognized in all erythroblasts in severe cases but only in haemoglobinized or polychromatic erythroblasts in early cases. The cells are larger than normal and the coarse chromatin of the normal normoblast nucleus is replaced by a more finely strippled chromatin.

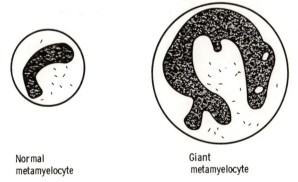

Normal
metamyelocyte

Giant
metamyelocyte

Fig. 12.4 Giant metamyelocyte.

Giant metamyelocytes are present (Fig. 12.4). These are cells that have failed to complete mitosis after having doubled or attempted to double their DNA and are incapable of further development. The hypersegmented neutrophils in the blood arise from more normal looking precursors.

Iron deficiency or thalassaemia if present at the same time, may make recognition of megaloblastic changes more difficult. This occurs in patients who have had a gastrectomy and in pregnancy. If in doubt iron should be given and the marrow repeated thereafter. Uncertain or equivocal marrow changes must be ignored. They are unlikely to be responsible for the patients symptoms or to be of any importance and merely mislead the physician attempting to reach an overall diagnosis.

Diagnosis of vitamin B$_{12}$ deficiency

In vitamin B$_{12}$ deficiency, the serum vitamin B$_{12}$ level is abnormally low. Most patients will excrete an increased amount of methylmalonic acid in the urine after oral valine but the mildest cases (highest vitamin B$_{12}$ levels) will still be normal.

Administration of 2 μg vitamin B$_{12}$ by injection each day will produce a good reticulocyte response but will not do so if the patient has folate deficiency. Finally, all except patients with nutritional vitamin B$_{12}$ deficiency, are unable to absorb vitamin B$_{12}$ normally. The patients with nutritional vitamin B$_{12}$ deficiency will respond fully to between 2–10 μg vitamin B$_{12}$ given each day *by mouth.*

Diagnosis of folic-acid deficiency

In clinical practice the diagnosis of folic-acid deficiency is often made by eliminating lack of vitamin B$_{12}$ as the cause of the anaemia. Vitamin B$_{12}$ deficiency may be excluded if the serum vitamin B$_{12}$ level is normal or if the patient (other than vegetarians who may lack vitamin B$_{12}$ in their diets) absorbs vitamin B$_{12}$ normally. In addition, in folic-acid deficiency the serum and the red cell folate levels are abnormally low and the urinary excretion of formiminoglutamic acid after oral histidine is abnormally high. Treatment with 200 μg folate daily by mouth usually gives a good reticulocyte response only in folate-deficient patients, but not in those with vitamin B$_{12}$ deficiency.

Sometimes patients who have a megaloblastic anaemia *due to folic-acid deficiency* have a depressed level of serum vitamin B$_{12}$. These folate-deficient patients absorb vitamin B$_{12}$ normally (unlike patients with true vitamin B$_{12}$ deficiency) and when treated with folic acid, the level of vitamin B$_{12}$ in the plasma returns to normal within 10 days.

The deoxyuridine suppression test

Normal folate and B$_{12}$ function is needed for the utilization of deoxyuridine for DNA synthesis. A single carbon unit is transferred to deoxyuridine to form thymidine which in turn is used for DNA. This is the synthetic path. In addition preformed thymidine is also reused for DNA and this is called the salvage path. In this test marrow cells are incubated with deoxyuridine to allow the synthetic pathway to operate and thereafter tritium-labelled thymidine is added to supply any remaining requirements for thymidine. Normal marrow cells meet about 95 per cent of their thymidine requirements by methylating deoxyuridine and generally less than 10 per cent of the requirements are met by taking up preformed ³H-thymidine (Figure 12.5,b). A megaloblastic marrow is unable to methylate deoxyuridine at a normal rate and hence more than 10 per cent of the ³H-thymidine is used (Figure 12.5,c). The addition of vitamin B$_{12}$ to the incubation mixture partially corrects the defect in B$_{12}$ deficiency and folate corrects the defect in both B$_{12}$ and folate deficiency. The test provides a rapid means of determining the nature of the deficiency as well as characterizing a biochemical defect present in megaloblastic anaemia.

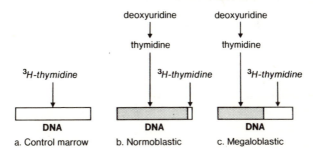

Fig. 12.5 Marrow cells are incubated with deoxyuridine. This is taken up by these cells, methylated to thymidine which in turn is incorporated into DNA. Less than 10 per cent of ³H-thymidine added later, is used for DNA synthesis (b). The control (a = 100 per cent uptake) is the uptake of ³H-thymidine alone. In megaloblastic marrow (c) due to impaired methylation of deoxyuridine because of B$_{12}$ or folate lack, less is used for DNA synthesis and more ³H-thymidine is used.

The haematological response

A proper response to treatment in megaloblastic anaemia is evidence that the correct haematinic has been given. Absence of response may mean a wrong diagnosis or interference with the response by infection, renal failure or complicating disease including cancer.

In an optimal response an adequate number of new red cells (reticulocytes) have been produced by the 5–7th day after starting treatment and the red cell count has increased significantly after the second week. The actual values depend on how anaemic the patient was at the start of treatment (day 0). If the red cell count was about 1 million/μl, 50 per cent of the cells may be reticulocytes on day 5 or 6. If the red cell count was 3 million/μl the corresponding figure may be only 4 or 5 per cent. Two types of response are illustrated (Fig. 12.6).

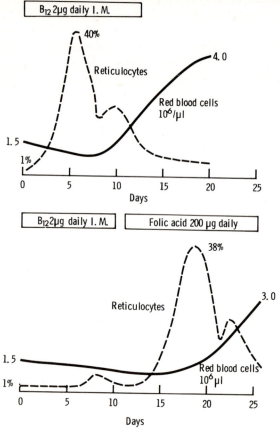

Fig. 12.6 The upper part of the Figure shows an optimal haematological response to treatment with vitamin B$_{12}$, the reticulocyte count showing the required rise on the 6th day after the start of treatment followed by a satisfactory increase in the red cell count. In the lower part of the Figure there is only a minor response to vitamin B$_{12}$ but a response to the correct haematinic, folic acid.

Biochemical changes in megaloblastic anaemia

In the untreated patient there is poor utilization of iron and the serum iron level tends to be high. The more anaemic the patient the higher is the serum iron level. Due to ineffective haemopoiesis, many cells fail to complete their development and die in the marrow. These dying cells release enzymes (lactic acid dehydrogenase and hydroxybutyric acid dehydrogenase) which attain very high levels in plasma. The mean red cell life span may be considerably reduced (20–30 days in severe cases), the plasma bilirubin level is raised (1–3 mg/100 ml), and urinary urobilinogen is increased. There may be evidence of associated or underlying disease such as excess fat in the stools (stearorrhoea).

Once successful treatment is instituted the serum iron and serum folate levels fall rapidly. There may be a small but generally insignificant fall in serum potassium. Figlu and MMA excretion fall after 2–3 days and become normal in a week. The marrow becomes largely normoblastic after 36–48 hours but giant metamyelocytes remain until they are removed by macrophages after two weeks.

Causes of megaloblastic anaemia

Vitamin B_{12} lack

Dietary. Vitamin B_{12} lack occurs in Hindu vegetarians who generally do not take milk, eggs nor meat in any form, but only have food of vegetable origin. Vitamin B_{12} is not present in the plant kingdom and hence the dietary vitamin B_{12} intake of vegetarians is very low.

Gastric causes. Intrinsic factor is needed for vitamin B_{12} absorption and this is normally produced by the parietal cells of the stomach. Gastric atrophy may lead to pernicious anaemia. Surgery on the stomach (gastrectomy) may lead to loss of the intrinsic-factor-secreting body of the stomach. There may be congenital absence of normal intrinsic factor.

Intestinal causes. The small gut is normally sterile and does not have any bacteria other than transient organisms entering from the mouth or via the ileo-caecal value. If a permanent bacterial population appears in the small gut the bacteria will abstract vitamin B_{12} from the food. Bacterial colonization is encouraged by loss of normal gut movement. Conditions in which bacteria can grow are the presence of intestinal blind loops or sacs, gut strictures, anastomoses (bits of gut joined together by inflammation or by the surgeon) and drugs that slow up gut movements.

Disease of the gut wall (regional ileitis, gluten-sensitive enteropathy, tropical sprue) may damage the vitamin B_{12} absorbing area of the ileum. Ileum may be excised surgically.

Folate lack

Increased requirements. Increased cell turnover increases the need for folate, for example, in pregnancy (and especially twin pregnancy), in haemolytic anaemia, in patients with rapidly growing tumours, generalized skin disorders etc. Ineffective haemopoiesis as in myelofibrosis, also leads to an increased need for folate.

Dietary. Folic acid is readily destroyed by light and heat—as in cooking. Inadequate amounts of poor quality food will not contain enough folate. Nutritional folate deficiency is found in old people and others on inadequate incomes. Premature babies have low folate stores. Their milk feeds may lose folate as a result of heating and folate deficiency may result.

Malabsorption of food folate may occur in coeliac disease due to sensitivity to wheat flour or in tropical sprue.

Other causes. Excessive alcohol when combined with an inadequate diet and drugs used in treating epilepsy (diphenylhydantoin or epanutin, primidone, barbiturates) are associated with folate deficiency.

Clinical aspects

Most patients with megaloblastic anaemia present with signs and symptoms of anaemia (Ch. 10). Others may complain of a sore mouth and/or tongue. Patients with vitamin B_{12} deficiency may also show abnormalities of the nervous system. They may have pins and needles sensation of both feet or/and hands (peripheral neuropathy). In addition they may have difficulty with walking, occasionally difficulty in urination, visual problems and rarely a strange variety of symptoms from unpleasant smells to hallucinations. These changes are called subacute combined degeneration of the cord. The nerve involvement disappears on vitamin B_{12} treatment although long-standing permanent damage to nerve cells is not reversed.

Pernicious anaemia

This is a disease of older people. It is due to atrophy of the stomach. There is loss of the normal secreting cells from the stomach mucosa and hence loss of intrinsic factor and of hydrochloric acid from the gastric juice.

Most of the patients come to their doctor because of tiredness, loss of energy and shortness of breath. A quarter have a sore mouth or tongue and a similar number have a tingling sensation in their limbs (paraesthesia). One third give a family history of this disease. It affects people of North European ancestry more often than other people.

The blood picture and marrow changes have been described. It is due to vitamin B_{12} deficiency, the serum vitamin B_{12} level is low and these patients cannot absorb vitamin B_{12}. Having taken steps to establish that such a patient has a megaloblastic anaemia due to vitamin B_{12} deficiency, the diagnosis of pernicious anaemia depends on the additional demonstration that intrinsic factor is absent from the gastric secretion. This may be done directly or indirectly.

1. There is failure to absorb oral labelled vitamin B_{12}. The absorption defect is corrected by giving the labelled vitamin B_{12} with extra intrinsic factor. This proves intrinsic factor lack.

2. The gastric juice may be examined. Both hydrochloric acid and intrinsic factor are absent.

Autoimmunity and pernicious anaemia. Pernicious anaemia is one of a group of diseases where the patient makes antibodies against some of his own tissues. This tendency is inherited so that among the patient's relatives there is an increased incidence of pernicious anaemia and sera from the patient's relatives often have gastric and thyroid antibodies even in the absence of clinical disease. These 'autoimmune' diseases tend to occur together in the same person. These conditions are pernicous anaemia, thyroid disease, atrophy of adrenal and atrophy of parathyroid glands.

In pernicious anaemia the patient makes humoral antibodies against gastric parietal cells (present in serum in 80–90 per cent) and against intrinsic factor (present in serum in 57 per cent). The pernicious anaemia patient also makes thyroid antibodies (present in serum in 25 per cent) and rather less commonly adrenal and parathyroid antibodies.

The parietal-cell antibody also occurs in about 5 per cent of the general population and the antibody prevents normal renewal of gastric mucosal cells so that gastric atrophy develops. The intrinsic-factor antibody combines with intrinsic factor and prevents it taking up vitamin B_{12}. By neutralizing the remaining intrinsic factor the antibody converts a low but adequate amount of secretion to an inadequate secretion so that severe malabsorption of vitamin B_{12} follows. Intrinsic-factor antibody is found only rarely apart from pernicious anaemia.

In addition to humoral antibodies, patients with pernicious anaemia have cell-mediated immunity against intrinsic factor. Positive migration-inhibition tests and transformation of pernicious-anaemia lymphocytes in presence of intrinsic factor are demonstrable in 80 per cent of patients.

Management in pernicious anaemia. Treatment with vitamin B_{12} which must be given by injection, restores the blood picture. There is a remarkable restoration of appetite and feeling of well-being within 48 hours. Thereafter adequate treatment is 250 μg hydroxocobalamin every second month carried on for the duration of the patients life. Hydroxocobalamin is given rather than cyanocobalamin because the former is much better retained in the body.

Eventually some 6 per cent of patients die with a cancer of the stomach.

Gastrectomy

Total gastrectomy usually carried out for cancer of the stomach, is accompanied by a cessation of vitamin B_{12} absorption. Regular

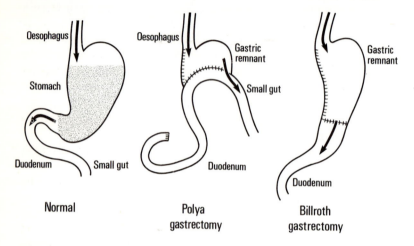

Fig. 12.7 The shaded area is normally removed in a partial gastrectomy. The upper end of the stomach that remains may then be joined to a loop of jejunum (Polya) or to the far end of the duodenum (Billroth 1).

injections of vitamin B_{12} are started after the operation. In those patients in whom the cancer has not spread outside the stomach, and who have not been given vitamin B_{12}, megaloblastic anaemia due to vitamin B_{12} deficiency appears after two to ten years.

Partial gastrectomy was carried out widely as treatment for gastric or duodenal ulceration. Nowadays it has been superceded by other operations (vagotomy and pyloroplasty). A high gastrectomy removes the part of the stomach shown as the shaded area in Figure 12.7. Continuity may be restored either by bringing up a loop of small gut and stitching it to the gastric remnant (polya gastrectomy), or by restoring continuity as in the Billroth operation (Fig. 12.7. The direction of 'food' flow is shown by the arrow.

Iron-deficiency anaemia develops in 50 per cent of post-gastrectomy patients after five years. This is due to poor absorption of food iron because the normal release of liquified food (chyme) from the stomach no longer operates and there is rapid passage of food down the gut. Secondly, the important iron-absorbing area in the upper gut is bypassed in the polya operation and left as a blind loop.

Generally the gastric remnant continues to secrete some acid and intrinsic factor. In others the mucosa of the remnant atrophies and intrinsic factor secretion declines. In fact about one third of patients do not absorb vitamin B_{12} normally after the operation and eventually 5 per cent get a megaloblastic anaemia due to vitamin B_{12} deficiency. Often the megaloblastic anaemia is accompanied by iron deficiency.

A further complication is the development of a permanent bacterial flora in the afferent loop left after a polya operation. When this occurs vitamin B_{12} absorption can be impaired not only because of lack of intrinsic factor but also because the bacteria take up both the vitamin B_{12} and the vitamin B_{12}-intrinsic factor complex.

Management. Because of the likelihood of anaemia appearing in half the patients who have undergone a partial gastrectomy, blood checks should be carried out once a year. Ideally this should include a blood count, serum iron and serum vitamin B_{12} estimation. Iron-deficiency is diagnosed in the usual way. If the serum vitamin B_{12} is low, a vitamin B_{12} absorption is done. If this is impaired monthly vitamin B_{12} injections are recommended.

It must not be forgotten that iron-deficiency anaemia can make recognition of megaloblastic changes difficult and even lead to a depression of the serum vitamin B_{12} level. It is often desirable to treat the iron-deficiency anaemia first and thereafter to assess vitamin B_{12} status.

Nutritional vitamin B_{12} deficiency

This is common among Hindu vegetarians and frequently leads to a megaloblastic anaemia. Proof of the diagnosis is a response to vitamin B_{12} given *by mouth*. The majority of strict vegetarians have low serum vitamin B_{12} levels and very much reduced stores of vitamin B_{12}. Most of these people are perfectly healthy. Only a minority develop megaloblastic anaemia. They should be encouraged to eat vitamin B_{12} containing foods. Treatment is to give several injections of hydroxo-cobalamin to restore vitamin B_{12} stores.

Childhood vitamin B_{12} deficiency

There are a number of rare disorders giving a severe megaloblastic anaemia at the end of the first or in the second year of life. A brother or sister may have the same disease and, sometimes, the parents are related suggesting that the gene responsible is transmitted in a recessive manner.

Congenital intrinsic-factor deficiency. There is no detectable intrinsic factor in the gastric juice. Otherwise the stomach is normal in all respects. Presumably the intrinsic factor molecule is abnormal and in one patient it was actually shown to react with an intrinsic-factor antibody although it was unable to promote vitamin B_{12} absorption. These children have a macrocytic anaemia and a megaloblastic marrow. As in pernicious anaemia they absorb vitamin B_{12} when normal intrinsic factor is added. They must be given vitamin B_{12} injections for life.

Congenital malabsorption of vitamin B_{12}. Here the stomach is normal and the gastric juice has a normal amount of intrinsic factor. These children differ from the children in the previous section in that they cannot absorb vitamin B_{12} at all. The defect lies in a failure of the distal small gut (ileum) to take up vitamin B_{12}. These children also have protein in the urine. Clinically they get a megaloblastic anaemia responding only to injections of vitamin B_{12} and these injections too must be continued for life.

Transcobalamin II deficiency. Absence of the B_{12} transport protein makes it impossible to carry B_{12} into cells or absorb it from the gut. Maternal TCII is available *in utero* but within a few months of birth severe megaloblastic anaemia develops. Vitamin B_{12} is still present on B_{12}-R binders in plasma (transcobalamin I), which normally accounts for most of the native B_{12} in plasma. However because TCII is lacking, the patient is unable to transport his own plasma-bound B_{12} into cells. Hence despite B_{12} deficiency the serum B_{12} level remains normal. Inheritance is recessive and parents have half the amount of TCII in their plasmas as compared to healthy subjects. Treatment is with injections of large amounts of B_{12} given every few days, so that some is able to diffuse into cells even in the absence of TCII.

Nutritional folate deficiency

Inadequate amount of poor quality food, or lack of desire to prepare and purchase food, is the cause of dietary lack of folate. Three groups of the population are more at risk—the very young, the very old and pregnant women.

Folic acid in food is preserved by reducing agents such as natural vitamin C (ascorbic acid). In feeding premature infants it was the practice in some institutions to make up all the feeds for the day heating the milk in preparation. This removed the vitamin C. Before giving the milk it was reheated. This now destroyed the folate which had been protected by the ascorbate and not surprisingly, some premature infants developed a megaloblastic anaemia. Breast-fed infants have significantly higher serum and red cell folate levels than bottle-fed infants, indicating that they receive more folate.

Old people may take very inadequate diets and about 8 per cent in the UK have low red cell folates. But pernicious anaemia will occur in almost 1 per cent of this age group.

Pregnancy is a period of increased folate need but the women who become anaemic are those who are nutritionally inadequate both for iron and for folic acid (see later).

Nutritional deficiency also plays a major role in megaloblastic anaemia of alcoholism and scurvy.

Effect of anticonvulsant drugs

A severe megaloblastic anaemia is seen occasionally in treated epileptics. More commonly macrocytosis occurs in the absence of anaemia and the marrow shows early megaloblastic changes.

The drugs have a number of actions which when combined may lead to folate deficiency. (1) The drugs interfere with the incorporation of thymidine into DNA in human marrow. Cells that are unable to complete DNA synthesis die in the marrow. (2) Some workers have found marginally impaired absorption of folic acid. If so it can be due to interference with renewal of gut cells as in (1). (3) The drugs activate liver enzymes which may lead to increased utilization of folic acid. All three mechanisms will ultimately lead to folate deficiency. Treatment is to give folic acid and the anticonvulsant drug is continued at the required dose.

Pregnancy

In well nourished populations about a quarter of pregnant women show early megaloblastic changes in the marrow at the end of pregnancy, although there is nothing to be seen in blood except possibly mild iron deficiency. Well-developed megaloblastic anaemia is relatively unusual. In Africa and Asia a high proportion of women in pregnancy are anaemic and this is due to both iron deficiency and folic-acid deficiency.

Folic-acid lack in pregnancy arises from two causes:

1. Inadequate dietary intake and inadequate body stores of folate. The women who get megaloblastic anaemia have lower serum and red cell folate levels at the beginning of pregnancy than those women who have an uncomplicated pregnancy.

2. There is an increased requirement for folic acid due to rapid

growth of the uterus, placenta and fetus. If there is twin pregnancy there is tenfold higher incidence of megaloblastic anaemia.

The diagnosis is made in the usual way by finding macrocytosis and a megaloblastic marrow either in the last few weeks of pregnancy in half the patients or in the puerperium in the remaining patients. The megaloblastosis is always due to folic-acid deficiency. Macrocytosis is a normal development in pregnancy provided enough iron is available. On the average the physiological increase in MCV is 4 fl but some healthy women show a much greater increase than this which must not be interpreted as due to megaloblastic haemopoiesis. Thus a marrow is essential for the diagnosis of megaloblastic anaemia in pregnancy. Anaemia in pregnancy is prevented by supplements containing not less than 200 μg folic acid daily and not less than 30 mg elemental iron (Ch. 19).

Haemolytic anaemia

The shortening of the mean red cell life span is accompanied by increased regeneration of blood. This increased turnover of red blood cells necessitates an increased supply of folic acid. Folic-acid lack may arise in chronic haemolytic disorders such as sickle-cell anaemia, untreated hereditary spherocytosis or long standing uncontrolled acquired haemolytic anaemia.

One should suspect megaloblastosis if a patient with haemolytic anaemia fails to maintain his or her expected reticulocyte level and becomes anaemic. Secondly, one should suspect megaloblastosis if such a patient starts needing blood transfusions to maintain an adequate haemoglobin level. Both these circumstances imply marrow failure and marrow aspiration is done to confirm the diagnosis. Patients with uncomplicated haemolytic anaemia often have a raised MCV but the presence of hypersegmented neutrophils would favour a megaloblastic process.

Often an additional 'folate stress' may arise, the commonest being pregnancy in women. Thus megaloblastic anaemia is common in women with a major haemoglobin disorder (SS. SC, Sthal disease) who become pregnant. Under these circumstances they become megaloblastic as early as the 20–25 week instead of near term as in uncomplicated pregnancy.

Treatment again is by oral folic acid.

Alcohol

Ethyl alcohol when taken in excess as in alcoholic drinks is a cell toxin. It damages a wide variety of tissues directly, including the marrow. In marrow spreads this can be recognized by mild megaloblastic changes, by ringed sideroblasts on Perl's stain and by excessive vacuolation particularly in early erythroblasts. These changes are present in various combinations in about half of exceptionally severe alcoholics and disappear within a few days of alcohol withdrawal. Less severe alcoholics only rarely show these severe toxic changes.

The effect on the peripheral blood of chronic alcoholic consumption is to produce a macrocytosis in the absence of anaemia and this is present in over 80 per cent of chronic alcoholics. In addition acute alcohol overdosage may lead to transient pancytopenia. The majority of alcoholics who are not anaemic have normal serum and red cell folate levels. Cessation of drinking results in a 'spontaneous' reticulocytosis and, if any of the elements are depressed, may be followed by a rise in haemoglobin, white cells and/or platelets.

Permanent megaloblastosis is not due to alcohol itself but is the result of long-standing associated nutritional folic-acid deficiency and responds to folic acid. This occurs in spirit and wine drinkers who do not take normal meals and is seen less often in beer drinkers since beer contains significant amounts of folic acid.

Chronic myelofibrosis

This disorder produces a characteristic blood picture with red and white cell precursors (including myeloblasts) in the blood, a relatively high platelet count and pear-shaped red cells. The patient often has an enormously enlarged spleen. There is a lot of unsuccessful haemopoiesis with death of cells in the marrow and spleen (where blood is also being made). This results in an increased requirement for folate.

Marrow failure may be indicated by the development of anaemia, a need for repeated blood transfusions or falling platelet count and this may be due in turn to folic-acid deficiency. Megaloblasts may be seen in buffy-coat preparations. Because of fibrosis of marrow it may be impossible to aspirate adequate material although strong suction may yield some fluid which, when spread, contains marrow cells.

Treatment is with folic acid.

13

Disorders of red blood cells

Haemolytic anaemia: Ineffective haemopoiesis:
Haemoglobinopathies: Sideroblastic anaemia.

Haemolytic anaemia

Normally red blood cells survive in the circulation for about 110 days. In these disorders their life span is shortened to only a few days in severe cases, to 10 or 20 days in milder ones. If the marrow is able to make up for the excessive loss of red cells by increased production there is no anaemia; if not, anaemia results. It is important to understand clearly the features that indicate excess destruction of red cells on the one hand, and regeneration by the marrow on the other. Both together give the picture seen in haemolytic anaemia.

Evidence of increased haemolysis

Bilirubin is the end product of haem break-down and accumulates with excessive red cell destruction. Clinically the patient may be jaundiced and the serum bilirubin level is usually between 1–3 mg/100 ml (17–50 μmol/l). The plasma generally appears yellow (icteric). The bilirubin is of the indirect (unconjugated) type. The urine may be dark but it does not contain bile (that is, there is an acholuric jaundice). It does, however, contain an increased amount of urobilinogen (Ch. 3).

Haptoglobins which are concerned in binding of free haemoglobin, are consumed and hence their level is reduced in the mildest cases and absent in the rest. Severe intravascular haemolysis may even result in free haemoglobin in plasma and hence some excretion of free haemoglobin in urine. Breakdown of free haemoglobin releases haem which when bound to albumin (methaemalbumin) is detected in the Schumm's test. With free haemoglobin in plasma and its excretion into urine, the test for blood in urine is positive despite absence of red cells on microscopy. The urine deposit may give a strongly positive reaction with Perls's stain, due to haemoglobin reabsorbed by the kidney tubules and appearing in casts in the urine.

Less direct evidence of haemolysis may be inferred from the appearance of the stained blood film which may show spherocytosis, abnormally-crenated red cells, red cell fragments or agglutination.

Finally, the increased red cell destruction may be measured by the reduced mean red cell life span using ^{51}Cr as a label. Surface counting may then indicate where these red cells are being destroyed, primarily the spleen or equally in spleen and liver.

Evidence of increased regeneration of red cells
This is indicated by an increase in new red cells, that is, an increased reticulocyte count. In the stained film this is shown as increased polychromasia. The marrow is of increased cellularity with erythroblasts predominating.

Classification of the haemolytic anaemias
The basic subdivision is between those disorders that are transmitted genetically (congenital) and those that are acquired. The latter are further grouped into antibody-produced (autoimmune) and others.

Congenital haemolytic anaemia: (1) Red cell membrane defects—hereditary spherocytosis. (2) Red cell enzymatic defects—for example, glucose-6-phosphate dehydrogenase and pyruvate kinase deficiency. (3) Haemoglobin defects—thalassaemias; aminoacid substitutions or deletions.

Acquired haemolytic anaemia: (4) Antibody induced—haemolytic disease of the newborn; autoimmune haemolytic anaemia; haemolytic anaemia due to high titre cold agglutinins; haemolytic anaemia due to drug-induced antibody reactions. (5) Mechanical damage as part of disseminated intravascular coagulation (DIC) or artificial heart valve. (6) Infections—malaria, Clostridium welchii. (7) Others—burns, hypersplenism, vitamin E deficiency. (8) Drugs—such as dapsone.

Investigation of a haemolytic anaemia
History is of great importance. Is there a family history of jaundice or of splenectomy? Are the parents related (recessive genes)? What is the racial origin of the patient? Haemoglobinopathies (S and C) are common in West Africans, Hb E in Thais and Chinese, thalassaemias are frequent in Mediterranean peoples, Indians and Chinese. Is the patient taking any medicine? Methyldopa used to treat raised blood pressure gives a haemolytic anaemia. Many drugs precipitate haemolytic anaemia if there is G6PD deficiency.

Attacks of abdominal pain due to gallstone colic is common in long standing cases because of excessive excretion of bile pigments which precipitate as pigment stones in the bile ducts and gall bladder.

Examination. Is the patient jaundiced? Does the urine contain urobilinogen? An enlarged spleen is frequent in haemolytic anaemia. Enlarged lymph glands may suggest underlying chronic lymphocytic leukaemia or lymphoma. Skin lesions and proteinuria may suggest disseminated lupus erythematosus (DLE) which may be associated with haemolytic anaemia.

Blood count. Cold agglutinins may be noted by agglutination of blood on the side of the blood count bottle. The MCV is raised in many haemolytic states due to a high proportion of young cells but the MCV may be low in alpha- and beta- thalassaemia syndromes and perhaps other haemoglobinopathies when they are associated with alpha-thalassaemia. Reticulocytosis is always present unless there is marrow failure. The level may be 3–4 per cent in the mildest cases to 20–60 per cent in severe ones. Acute haemolysis may be accompanied by a leucocytosis.

The red cells in the blood film will show polychromasia and in addition may show spherocytosis, fragmentation, elliptocytes, agglutinates or malarial parasites. There may be an associated but significant disorder like glandular fever or chronic lymphocytic leukaemia.

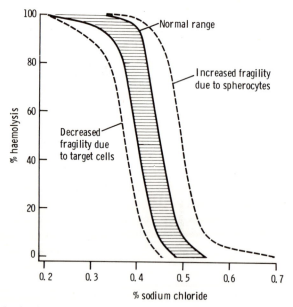

Fig. 13.1 Lysis of red cells in hypotonic saline. The normal range is indicated. Increased fragility of spherocytic red cells is shown in the result to the right of the normal range. Flattened red cells are more resistant than normal to haemolysis and appear as the result to the left of the normal range.

Osmotic fragility tests. The rounder the red cell the more readily does it lyse in low salt concentrations. This test may confirm the presence of spherocytes noted on the film or may help when the appearance of the film is equivocal. Note that normally there is less than 5 per cent haemolysis in 0·5 per cent NaCl. (Fig. 13.1) Incubation of the blood for 24 hours stresses these cells metabolically and accentuates mild spherocytic changes.

Autohaemolysis test. When red cells are incubated at 37°C a small number haemolyse with release of haemoglobin. In hereditary spherocytes, not only do the red cells lyse more readily, but haemolysis is largely prevented by the addition of glucose.

Serology

The antiglobulin test. This test is used to detect 'incomplete' antibodies that do not cause direct agglutination of red cells. When such an antibody is already present on the red cell surface the antiglobulin serum will cause such cells to agglutinate (direct antiglobulin test). If the antibody is in serum, red cells may be added and after incubation tested with the antiglobulin serum to see if the red cells have taken up the antibody (indirect antiglobulin test). The antiglobulin reagent should react with IgG immunoglobulins and also with IgM immunoglobulins. IgM antibodies generally produce agglutination, but occasionally when relatively few molecules attach to each red cell this may not happen. Red cells which have reacted with IgM, however, almost invariably bind complement components and these complement components are detected with the antiglobulin serum. Monospecific antiglobulin sera are available that react with IgG, IgA, IgM, and C_3 and C_4 components of complement only.

Antibody on the red cell surface in haemolytic anaemia is detected with the antiglobulin test and the use of monospecific antisera will identify the type of immunoglobulin or complement. The antibody can be eluted from the red cell surface by heat and its characteristics tested. These are two types:

Warm antibodies	*Cold antibodies*
Usually IgG	Usually IgM
Detected by antiglobulin test.	Generally directly agglutinating.
React between 0–37°C.	React best in cold.
Rarely fix complement.	Always fix complement.
Often have Rhesus specificity.	Usually anti-I, rarely anti-i.

Serum antibody. Free antibodies in serum are usually of the cold type with anti-I specificity and may be of very high titre. They fix complement and hence cause haemolysis. Clinically their thermal amplitude, that is, the highest temperature at which they react with red cells, is important. Antibodies only active at 3–6°C are of little importance but those which are active at normal skin temperature (about 31°C) can lead to destruction of red cells in the body and hence to a haemolytic anaemia.

Enzymes. Haemolytic anaemia occurs in patients whose red cells lack certain glycolytic enzymes. The most important are glucose-6-phosphate dehydrogenase and pyruvate kinase. Screening tests and direct assays are available for both these enzymes. Significant deficiencies of other enzymes are exceedingly rare.

Heinz bodies. These consist of precipitated globin chains of haemoglobin and they are visualized by incubating the blood with methyl violet or brilliant cresyl blue when the purple dye is taken up by the precipitated globin. They occur when there is defective reducing capacity in the cell as in glucose-6-phosphate dehydrogenase deficiency and particularly after drugs which stress this pathway. This may lead to oxidation of the haemoglobin and precipitation of globin. It also occurs when there is an unstable haemoglobin. The spleen will remove red cells containing abnormal particles from the circulation but after splenectomy, they persist in the blood. *In vitro*, a blood sample can be incubated with acetylphenylhydrazine and large numbers of Heinz bodies will be produced if reducing pathways are deficient.

Other tests. Ham's test, sugar lysis test, haemoglobin electrophoresis, haemoglobin heat stability test, oxygen-dissociation curves and screening for disseminated intravascular coagulation may be required in the investigation of a patient with haemolytic anaemia.

General approach

Is there haemolysis? A persistently elevated reticulocyte count not explained in other ways favours haemolysis but an undiagnosed major gastrointestinal bleed can have a similar effect. The mildest cases will have normal bilirubin levels but haptoglobins will usually be absent.

What does the blood film show? It may be spherocytic, non-spherocytic, show agglutination or more bizarre features. If the film shows spherocytes and the direct antiglobin test is negative, the diagnosis is probably hereditary spherocytosis. If the blood film is spherocytic and there is a positive antiglobulin test there is an autoimmune haemolytic anaemia (idiopathic, methyldopa, chronic lymphocytic leukaemia, lymphoma). Agglutinates in the stained peripheral blood film suggests cold antibody haemolytic anaemia due to anti-I. Where the antiglobulin test is negative and the film is not spherocytic but there is evidence of haemolysis, a wider range of investigations are required. These include haemoglobin electrophoresis, heat stability tests, glucose-6-phosphate dehydrogenase and pyruvate kinase tests, Ham's test etc., the precise approach being suggested by the racial background of the patient, age, family history, etc.

Hereditary spherocytosis
This disease is familial being transmitted as a dominant characteristic. Other members of the family may have had their spleens removed and a history of this may extend over several generations. A third of patients do not have a family history—? mutation of a gene. It is the commonest congenital haemolytic anaemia in Northern Europe.

The patient may present as jaundice in the newborn or with jaundice in later life. He or she may complain of tiredness if anaemic, leg ulcers, gall stone colic due to formation of pigment gallstones or very severe anaemia due to an aplastic crisis. It is not known why such patients (and others with chronic haemolysis) are susceptible to chronic intractable leg ulcers. The spleen is usually enlarged.

There is probably a defect in the red cell membrane and an abnormal protein in the red cell membrane has been implicated. Whatever the basic disorder there is abnormal flux of sodium and potassium across the red cell membrane and thus the red cell in hereditary spherocytosis requires a lot of glucose to provide energy in order to retain potassium in the cell and to pump out excess sodium. When such a cell is delayed in the spleen it is cut off from its supply of glucose in the plasma and becomes metabolically abnormal. The reticulocytes in this disease appear normal and only older cells are spherocytic. It is supposed that in the spleen bits of the metabolically-abnormal cells are 'nipped off' as has been demonstrated with antibody-coated red cells and as a result the surface area to volume ratio changes so that the cell becomes more spherical. Such cells are eventually destroyed either in the spleen or elsewhere in the body.

The blood film shows spherocytes and the fragility test is abnormal. The MCHC is often increased to even as high as 37 per cent. Autohaemolysis is abnormal and improved significantly by glucose. There is a small increase in plasma bilirubin which is indirect reacting and an elevated faecal and urinary urobilinogen.

Aplastic crisis. The aplastic crisis is an episode of severe anaemia due to marrow failure often precipitated by trivial infections like a common cold. Haemopoiesis ceases and the marrow empties of all dividing cells. New cell lines start from stem cells. The effects on the patient are due to the resulting anaemia. In hereditary spherocytosis the mean red cell life span is between 10–20 days and the haemoglobin falls from 12–13 g/100 ml to 2–3 g eight to ten days later. When the haemogobin falls the patient begins to feel ill and thus he or she presents to the doctor with a very low haemoglobin concentration. At this time the marrow is well on the way to recovery being full of erythroblasts. Anaemia with spherocytes in the film accompanied by very low reticulocyte levels suggests aplastic arrest. In the early stages white cells and platelets are also reduced. Once the diagnosis is made no treatment may be needed but sometimes a transfusion is desirable to alleviate the effects of severe anaemia. Platelets and white cells recover sooner than red cells.

Similar aplastic arrests occur in normal subjects but because the red cells have a normal survival, temporary cessation of the supply of new red cells from the marrow merely causes the haemoglobin to drift down from 14 to 12 g. This is followed by recovery so that such cases are rarely noted clinically. An example of aplastic arrest complicating

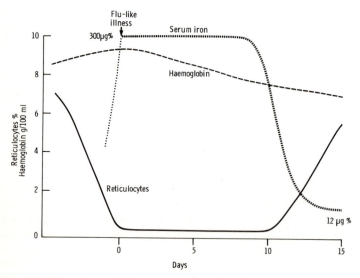

Fig. 13.2 This patient was being treated with oral iron for an iron-deficiency anaemia when he developed a 'flu-like' illness. Next day his reticulocyte count was found to be zero. The serum iron rose to a high level and the marrow lacked all red cell precursors. When recovery started there was a fall in the serum iron followed by re-appearance of reticulocytes. The haemoglobin level drifted down steadily over this period.

iron-deficiency anaemia is shown in Figure 13.2. Note the high serum iron level throughout the aplastic phase.

Hereditary spherocytosis is familial and if the infection affects other members of the family with hereditary spherocytosis, these too may suffer an aplastic arrest. Marrow failure can also be due to folate deficiency but this is commoner in SS disease.

Treatment. Treatment of hereditary spherocytosis is by splenectomy which removes the site where the red cell undergoes stasis and consequent damage. Clinically all cases are virtually cured although the cells remain spherocytic. The mean cell life after splenectomy remains slightly shortened (about 80 days). In children the operation should be postponed until the age of three if possible. Relapse is rare and is due to the presence of splenic tissue, either splenunculi overlooked at surgery, or autotransplants of splenic tissue.

Glucose-6-phosphate dehydrogenase deficiency

In 1956 a patient being treated for malaria with the drug primaquine had an acute haemolytic episode. This patient had very low levels of G6PD in his red cells and it was suggested that lack of the enzyme made the antimalarial drug (primaquine) so dangerous to this patient. It was then realized that the relatively common condition of favism, an acute haemolytic episode in children eating broad beans (*Vicia fava*) known in the Middle East for centuries, occurred only in G6PD-deficient children.

Deficiency of this enzyme occurs in many millions of people in West Africa, shores of the Mediterranean, Middle East and Far East. Deficiency is high in malarial areas suggesting that it provided some protection against malaria.

There are more than 50 types of G6PD enzymes which, like the abnormal haemoglobins, have aminoacid substitutions and hence different electrophoretic mobilities. The gene for G6PD is carried on the sex chromosome (X chromosome). Males (XY) are either normal or deficient having either a normal X or G6PD-deficient X from their mothers. In women (XX) who carry one G6PD deficient X (heterozygotes) half the red cells have a full G6PD complement and the other half virtually none. This is because in every cell in females one of the two X chromosomes is normally inactivated (Fig. 13.3). By chance this may be either the normal X or the G6PD defective X.

Glucose-6-phosphate is the entry point via the enzyme G6PD into the pentose-phosphate shunt which produces NADPH required for maintaining reduced glutathione (GSH) (Ch. 5). Under normal circumstances other reducing systems in the cell cope with converting

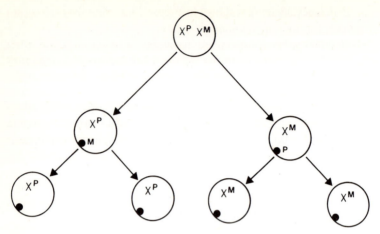

Fig. 13.3 One X chromosome in the female cell is derived from the father (X^P) and the other from the mother (X^M). One of these X chromosomes is inactivated and there is an equal likelihood that this is the X^P or X^M. Thereafter the progeny of this cell continue to replicate the same active X chromosome. The cells in a normal female are a mixture of these two types. A tumour arising from a single cell will only have X^P or X^M.

methaemoglobin to oxyhaemoglobin. When oxidant drugs are taken these remaining reducing systems are inadequate and without supplies of GSH, methaemoglobin accumulates and globin is oxidized to produce Heinz bodies which precipitate in the cell. The red cells are distorted and either removed by macrophages or lysed in the circulation. Deficiency of different types of enzymes have different clinical manifestations. The commonest type of G6PD has been designated 'B'. Among Africans another variant termed 'A' occurs and the most common variant among Caucasians has been called 'Mediterranean type'. Evidence for the clonal origin of some disorders such as chronic granulocytic leukaemia has been deduced from the presence of one of these variants only in 'tumour' cells whereas one or other is present in cells from other tissues such as skin. The defect is fully expressed in affected males. Female heterozygotes have two populations of red cells, one deficient in G6PD, the other normal. The proportion of affected cells vary considerably in different individuals so that some affected females appear to be virtually normal and others fully affected.

Clinically G6PD deficiency may present as jaundice in the new born even requiring exchange transfusion with the risk of Kernicterus (brain damage), as attacks of acute haemolysis or as a chronic non-spherocytic haemolytic anaemia. Some cases come to notice as the result of investigation of unexplained macrocytosis.

In a G6PD-deficient subject an attack may commence three days after starting the drug with jaundice, anaemia and haemoglobin in the urine (Fig. 13.4). There is a reticulocytosis, Heinz bodies and red cell fragments in the film. Nevertheless although the drug is continued the episode is self-limiting. This is because only older red cells with very low G6PD levels are susceptible. As these cells are replaced by young cells (with somewhat more G6PD) they are no longer susceptible to the oxidant action of the drug. Many drugs have such actions

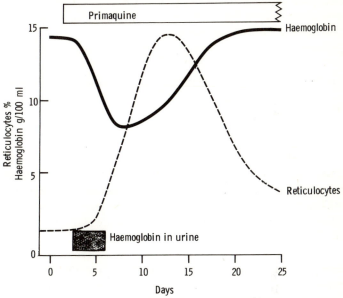

Fig. 13.4 Primaquine given to treat malaria in a G6PD deficient subject caused acute haemolysis with fall in haemoglobin and appearance of free haemoglobin in urine. There is a reticulocytosis. Despite continuing the drug haemolysis stops because the new red cells are more resistant to the drug.

including antimalarials (Primaquine, Chloroquine), Sulphonamides, antibiotics (Penicillin, Streptomycin), antibacterials (Nitrofurantoin) and salicylates (Aspirin). Products of broad beans enjoyed by millions of children, can precipitate a similar episode. A febrile illness may also precipitate a haemolytic episode.

Pyruvate-kinase deficiency
Lack of this enzyme reduces the utilization of glucose for producing ATP in the red cell. The disorder is rare and transmitted as a recessive characteristic. The patient is usually a child, anaemia is variable in

degree, there is splenomegaly and the blood picture is that of a non-spherocytic haemolytic anaemia. The only diagnostic test is the assay of the enzyme level in the red cells.

Methaemoglobinaemia

The oxidized form of haemoglobin is methaemoglobin. A raised level of methaemoglobin in blood may result from abnormal haemoglobins (collectively called Haemoglobins M). In these disorders (Hb Boston, Saskatoon, Iwate, Hyde Park and Milwaukee) an amino acid substitution allows an extra electron to reach the iron atom so that it becomes oxidized to Fe^{+++} instead of Fe^{++}. These patients tend to be polycythaemic rather than anaemic.

Secondly, methaemoglobinaemia can be due to chronic eating of drugs like phenacetin and thirdly, to lack of an enzyme called methaemoglobin reductase (Ch. 5). Apart from a blue discoloration of the skin (cyanosis) in those patients with about 20 per cent methaemoglobin, these patients are well.

Paroxysmal nocturnal haemoglobinuria

This is a rare acquired haemolytic anaemia wherein the red cells are prematurely broken up in the circulation with appearance of haemoglobin in the urine. Haemolysis often occurs at night, the early morning urine being very dark. Although there may be a very marked reticulocytosis in some patients the mean cell life may be so shortened that transfusion is needed. Many drugs aggravate the condition. The blood film is unremarkable and it is another example of a non-spherocytic haemolytic anaemia. The diagnostic test is the small amount of lysis of the patients red cells produced by acidified serum (Ham's test) and latterly the sugar lysis test has also been used.

A positive Ham's test rarely occurs in hypoplastic anaemia and in dyserythropoietic anaemia with multinucleated normoblasts.

Autoimmune haemolytic anaemia

This is usually a spherocytic haemolytic anaemia with a positive direct antiglobulin test. A 1000 bed hospital may expect to see one or two such cases per year. The patient presents with anaemia or jaundice. It occurs at all ages.

In about half the cases of autoimmune haemolytic anaemia no underlying cause is detectable. In the remainder a tumour of lymph glands is present (lymphoma) or chronic lymphatic leukaemia may be present. It may be part of disseminated lupus erythematosus (DLE) or be associated with other drugs such as methyldopa (Aldomet) used to treat raised blood pressure. Rarely an ovarian tumour or thymoma may be present. Other autoimmune diseases may be present including thyroid disease, pernicious anaemia, thrombocytopenia etc. In a survey of over 200 patients 52 per cent had an enlarged spleen, 45 per cent an enlarged liver, 34 per cent lymphadenopathy, 21 per cent were jaundiced but only 4 per cent showed pallor.

The nature of the antibody coating the red cells has been described. The antibody can be eluted from red cells and sometimes has some specificity within the Rh system.

Management. Management consists of measures to reduce antibody production and to reduce excessive destruction of red cells. The standby is steroids in very large doses if necessary, in the first instance. To these may be added immunosuppressive drugs such as cyclophosphamide or azathiaprine (Imuran). Transfusion should be avoided but may have to be given if the haemoglobin level falls too rapidly.

If after labelling red cells with ^{51}Cr there is evidence on surface counting that the spleen is playing a dominant role in destroying red cells, splenectomy is likely to prove beneficial but this should be done only if steroids and other drugs fail. The operation carries a significant mortality and post-operative thrombotic complications due to a high platelet count can be formidable.

Cases associated with methyldopa are of special interest. This drug induces an autoimmune haemolytic, although the drug itself appears to play no direct role in the antigen-antibody reaction. Twenty per cent of patients on this drug in time get a positive direct antiglobulin test but only 1 in 200 patients get a full blown haemolytic anaemia. Withdrawal of methyldopa alone controls haemolysis after 2–3 months and the antiglobulin test eventually becomes negative after 1–2 years. How the drug stimulates the development of autoimmune haemolytic anaemia is not known.

Haemolytic anaemia due to cold agglutinins
Many normal sera contain cold agglutinins of low titre (up to 1 in 32) and detectable at low temperature (4 to 10°C). Occasionally a patient develops a cold antibody in high titre (more than 1 in 1000) which is active at relatively high temperatures (greater than 20°C). This antibody reacts with all red blood cells from adults but not with cord blood cells and hence is said to have anti-I specificity. The antibody is an IgM immunoglobulin. When attached to red cells the complex binds complement and is haemolytic.

Haemolytic anaemia due to high titre cold agglutinins is a relatively rare disorder—a large hospital may see a case every 2–3 years. The patient may have the signs and symptoms of anaemia. In addition on exposure to cold the patients develop numbness of the fingers, toes, nose and ears which acquire a white or blue cyanosed appearance (Raynaud's phenomenon). This is due to formation of clumps of red cells in small blood vessels with slowing of the circulation (stasis). Anaemia can be severe with haemoglobin levels of less than 6 g/100 ml and the reticulocyte level may not be very high (about 10 per cent) suggesting poor marrow response possibly because the antibody is also affecting developing erythroblasts. In very chronic cases the haemoglobin will tend to decline in winter and improve in summer. These chronic cases tend to be associated with a tumour of lymph glands (lymphoma) and they may respond to treatment with chlorambucil (2–4 mg/day). Other measures are avoidance of cold which may well mean the patient being indoors all winter.

Transient high titre cold agglutinins may occur after what was called 'primary atypical pneumonia'. This is now believed to be due to infection with *Mycoplasma pneumoniae* and characteristically the antibody (and haemolytic anaemia) appear 2–3 weeks after the respiratory infection. Rarely an anti-i antibody may produce a haemolytic anaemia as part of *glandular fever*.

A very rare disorder is *paroxymal cold haemoglobinuria*. Haemoglobin is passed in the urine following exposure to cold and may be accompanied by back pain and pyrexia. It was always said to be related to syphilis but also to virus infections (mumps, measles, chicken pox). The antibody (an IgG immunoglobulin) attaches to red blood cells in the cold (up to about 17°C in some cases) but lysis due to complement binding occurs in the warm. Patients must thus be severely chilled before they get an attack. The antibody only reacts with blood group P positive cells. The temperature requirements are used in the Donath-Landsteiner test for this antibody, only samples which are chilled reacting and showing lysis, whereas controls kept at 37°C fail to react.

Drug-induced immune haemolytic anaemia

Drugs may result in an immune haemolytic anaemia. The drug may bind very firmly to the red cell and an antibody is formed against the red cell-drug complex. This is the case with penicillin and cephalosporin (haptene mechanism).

A different mechanism is when an antibody is formed against a drug-plasma protein complex. The drug-protein complex absorbs on to red cells and then antibody and complement attach. This occurs with quinine and phenacetin (immune-complex formation).

A third mechanism has been mentioned in relation to Aldomet (methyldopa) which leads to an autoimmune haemolytic anaemia indistinguishable from the 'idiopathic' type. The drug does not take part in the immune reaction. It may be termed autoantibody induction.

Haemolytic anaemia occurring in a patient who is taking tablets or other forms of medication must raise the possibility that the drug is responsible. The red cells give a positive antiglobulin test. White cells and platelets may also be reduced in numbers. If a drug is implicated, then withdrawal of the drug should of itself produce haematological improvement within 10 days. If it is important that the patient receive the drug and its role in the anaemia is uncertain, cautious challenge of the patient with the drug may be justified.

Drug-induced haemolytic anaemia (non-immune)
Drugs may be oxidizing agents and lead to damage (denaturation) of haemoglobin which form Heinz bodies. This can occur with:

1. Normal red cells by drugs such as acetylphenylhydrazine, sulphones (Dapsone) and sodium chlorate.
2. Red cells with unstable haemoglobin (Hb Koln, Zurich, Saskatoon). The anaemia has also been called 'Heinz body anaemia'. Many drugs including sulphonamides may precipitate haemolysis but infection alone can also do so.
3. Red cells with enzyme deficiencies involving reducing systems such as G6PD deficiency and glutathione reductase deficiency.

Haemolytic anaemia due to mechanical damage to red cells
Red blood cells can be torn apart by mechanical trauma such as strands of fibrin across vessels, foreign fibres in artificial heart valves or acute physical pressures.

Disseminated intravascular coagulation associated with failure of kidney function results in abnormal deposition of fibrin and may lead to brisk intravascular destruction of red cells as the red cell is torn by being forced through a fibrin mesh. There is free haemoglobin in plasma and the blood film shows red-cells fragments (schistocytes). This has been called the haemolytic-uraemic syndrome or micro-angiopathic haemolytic anaemia.

Patients with artificial heart valves made of a material called teflon may develop a similar haemolytic anaemia due to red cells being torn by the mesh of fabric. This occurs if the valve has not been covered by a lining of endothelial tissue by the surgeon. Cure is effected by a further operation which covers these bare surfaces.

Long-distance runners (20–100 miles) regularly have a haemolytic anaemia at the end of a long run. The red cells are crushed by the pressure in the soles of their feet and is partly overcome by lining their shoes with soft material. Once again red cell fragments are present, serum haptoglobin is low or absent and urine may be red due to free haemoglobin. The condition is called March Haemoglobinuria following its recognition in soldiers after long route marches.

Other haemolytic anaemias

Malaria causes a haemolytic anaemia not only because cells containing parasites are destroyed but red cells not infested with malaria may be destroyed prematurely. The mechanism is uncertain. It has been suggested that breakdown products of the malarial parasite may absorb on to red cells and then react with a malarial antibody and complement. Positive direct antiglobulin tests have been recorded. Other patients do not have a positive antiglobulin test and a hyperactive spleen may damage the red cells. Drugs used to treat malaria may also produce haemolysis. A form of acute haemolysis in malaria has been termed 'blackwater fever'.

Bacteria such as Clostridium welchii may release a haemolysin giving rise to a haemolytic anaemia. Other organisms may act through septicaemia and disseminated intravascular coagulation. Certain *snake venoms* (cobra, viper) act on the red cell membrane (via a lysolecithin) and rarely produce a haemolytic anaemia. Severe *burns* may damage blood directly with marked sphering.

Ineffective haemopoiesis

In a number of blood diseases failure to produce enough blood is associated with the failure of developing cells in the marrow to mature into normal red cells. The precursor cells die in the marrow and are phagocytosed. This may arise because of lack of essential nutrients (vitamin B_{12}, folate, possibly iron), lack of enzyme systems that are needed for forming viable cells (congenital dyserthropoietic anaemias, thalassaemia, sideroblastic anaemia) or due to toxic substances (lead, possibly alcohol) or for less well understood reasons as in myelofibrosis. The term ineffective haemopoiesis describes this intramedullary failure of red cell production. The condition may be recognized by:

1. Association of a cellular erythroid marrow with anaemia as in untreated megaloblastic anaemia. The death of erythroblasts in the marrow causes release of enzymes such as lactic acid dehydrogenase and hydroxybutyrate dehydrogenase into plasma. Morphologically

these 'dead' erythroblasts are recognized by the deep blue basophilic staining of cytoplasm, by the separation of the cytoplasm from nucleus and loss of normal nuclear staining characteristics and their replacement by a bland uniform nuclear stain.

2. Poor incorporation of ^{59}Fe into red cells despite a normal or rapid plasma-iron clearance.

3. Early excretion in the faeces of haem breakdown products. Glycine is required for haem synthesis and glycine labelled with ^{15}N provides a cohort label (Ch. 2). Erythroblasts dying in the marrow will release synthesized haem which will then appear in faeces as stercobilin. Haem in red cells appears as stercobilin at the end of the life span of the red cells. The diagram (Fig. 13.5) shows that normally some 15 per cent of stercobilin appears within a week of

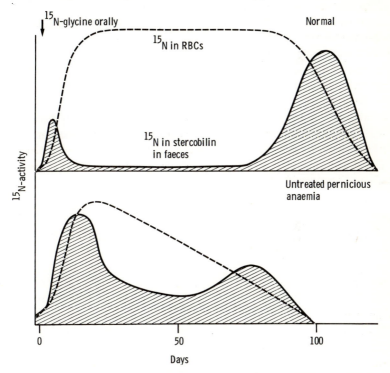

Fig. 13.5 ^{15}N-glycine serves as a cohort label for red cells. Normally some of the normoblasts fail to complete development and there is some excretion of ^{15}N as stercobilin in faeces (upper half of Figure). The bulk of ^{15}N appears at the end of the life span of the red cells. The lower half of the Figure shows what happens in ineffective haemopoiesis where there is considerable excretion of ^{15}N from defective erythroblasts in the first few days. The random destruction of red cells in pernicious anaemia results in a steady fall of the ^{15}N level in red cells.

giving the label due to failure of some cells to develop but most (85 per cent) appears at the end of the red cell life span. In ineffective haemopoiesis (as in untreated pernicious anaemia) the early stercobilin peak is much greater.

Haemoglobinopathies

Diseases affecting the globin part of haemoglobin fall into two groups. Firstly, where there is a substitution of a normal aminoacid in the polypeptide globin chain by another aminoacid and, secondly, where the rate of globin synthesis is sub-normal (thalassaemia).

The severity of the symptoms depend on whether the abnormality is inherited from only one parent (heterozygous) or from both parents (homozygous), and on the precise consequences of the lesion. These diseases are transmitted as dominant characteristics.

Most of the additional techniques that are required for investigation are within the scope of most laboratories. These are:

1. Evidence of a haemolytic anaemia. Target cells may be present in blood films and with this, an increased resistance of the red cells to haemolysis in hypotonic solution. Sickle cells may be present in the stained blood film and inclusion bodies such as Heinz bodies and Hb H inclusion bodies may be looked for under appropriate circumstances. For Hb H inclusions in α-thalassaemia the reticulocyte rich portion (top of the red cell column in a PCV tube) of a fresh blood sample is incubated for one hour with 1 per cent brilliant cresyl blue and a film examined without counterstaining.
2. The appearance of sickle cells under reducing conditions.
3. Estimation of fetal haemoglobin.
4. Electrophoresis of the haemolysate using either cellulose acetate, starch gel, starch block or polyacrylamide gel. The aminoacid substitution may change the net charge on the haemoglobin and hence change its electrophoretic mobility. Elution of the haemoglobin bands and measurement of their optical density provides a quantitative measure of the haemoglobin components including Hb A_2.
5. The heat denaturation test enables one to suspect an unstable haemoglobin which precipitates at 50°C.
6. The solubility test. Reduced Hb S is poorly soluble and this test is useful in distinguishing homozygous SS from heterozygous SD combinations.
7. Tryptic digestion of the isolated globin and identification of abnormal residues following chromatography of the digest (fingerprinting).

8. Incubation of reticulocyte-rich blood with ^{3}H-leucine leads to its incorporation into the globin chains. These may be isolated and normally as much isotope is incorporated into the α-chains as into all the others so that the ratio is 1. The ratio is greater than 1 if β-chain synthesis is depressed and less than 1 if α chain synthesis is depressed.

Haemoglobins S, C, D and E

By far the most important is Hb S because of its tendency to produce irreversibly sickled red cells. In all these conditions there is an aminoacid substitution in the β-globin chain.

Sickle cell anaemia (Hb SS).

The S gene is present in high frequency across tropical Africa. A low frequency is present in population groups in Cyprus, Greece, Middle East and India. S trait may afford some protection from malaria since the distribution of the S gene (and G6PD deficiency gene) and malaria coincide, that is, the malarial parasite is less successful in establishing itself in red cells with Hb S. This relative protection afforded to subjects with the S trait, because of a relative resistance to malaria, is called balanced polymorphism.

Uncomplicated SS disease is a severe haemolytic anaemia with a reduced haemoglobin concentration (6–10 g/100 ml) and an elevated reticulocyte count (15–40 per cent). Sickle cells may be seen in an ordinary blood film—a feature shared with S-thalassaemia. Adults usually lose their spleen as a result of thrombosis of the splenic blood vessels, and hence the blood film also shows Howell-Jolly bodies, many target cells and normoblasts. Haemoglobin electrophoresis shows that 80–95 per cent of the haemoglobin is Hb S and the remainder Hb F. The higher the Hb F content the milder the disease.

The abnormality is replacement of the 6th aminoacid in the β-polypeptide chain (normally glutamic acid) by valine. At low oxygen tension which may follow stagnation of blood in capillaries, Hb S may come out of solution as long filaments. The twisting of these filaments of crystalline globin gives rise to a rope-like appearance and an irreversibly sickled red cell. The tendency to sickling is hastened because Hb S gives up its oxygen relatively more easily than Hb A. At the same time, because of the relative ease in the transfer of oxygen, the patient has relatively good exercise tolerance despite relatively low haemoglobin levels.

The course of the disease is interrupted by series of crises.

Painful (infarctive) crisis. This may be due to blockage of small arteries and hence death of tissue (infarction). In small children the small bones of the hands may be involved (dactylitis), the heads of long bones, lungs or eye. It can present as acute abdominal pain or as painful persistent erection of the penis (priapism). Treatment of the sickle-cell crisis is by warmth, analgesics, measures to expand plasma volume, measures to deal with infection and measures to deal with disseminated intravascular coagulation. Some situations such as retinal vein thrombosis (and possible blindness) and priapism require more urgent measures such as streptokinase therapy or defibrination with substances like Arvin.

Sequestration crisis. This occurs particularly in young children and is characterized by a sudden massive pooling of blood largely in the spleen. There is severe anaemia and collapse. The outcome may be fatal.

Aplastic crisis. Here there is marrow failure and severe anaemia associated with minor infection as described earlier.

Megaloblastic crisis. Arrest of haemopoiesis is often due to severe folic-acid deficiency and a megaloblastic marrow. For this reason a marrow examination is essential. Treatment is with folic acid orally.

Haemolytic crisis. Perhaps as a result of infection the rate of haemolysis may be accelerated so that there is increased jaundice and increased anaemia. It may be part of an infarctive crisis but gallstones giving obstructive jaundice must be excluded.

Administration of folic acid regularly as a prophylactic measure is the rule. Infections should be treated promptly with antibiotics. Pregnancy is relatively dangerous in patients with homozygous sickle-cell disease with significant mortality. Folic acid and possibly regular transfusions of normal blood throughout pregnancy may be needed in those with a bad history.

Other complications in this disease are bony abnormalities of the sort described in thalassaemia. Infection in bone (osteomyelitis) with salmonella organisms may occur. Impaired renal function is common since infarctions with renal papillary necrosis occurs. Chronic leg ulcers are a common feature.

Sickle-cell trait (Hb SA). The heterozygote (Fig. 13.6) does not suffer any disability. The blood appears normal. They run some risk if given an anaesthetic gas mixture with low oxygen content or in unpressurized aircraft where the partial pressure of oxygen can also fall.

Sickle-cell-thalassaemia. This combination is often very difficult to distinguish from SS disease and family study may be required. One parent should have sickle-cell trait and the other thalassaemia trait.

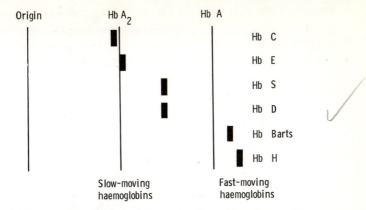

Fig. 13.6 Haemoglobin electrophoresis showing the position of some of the commoner types of haemoglobins.

Hb SC. These patients have a haemolytic anaemia with many of the features of SS disease but are less severely affected.

Others. Hb CC and Hb AC are relatively mild conditions, the blood film showing target cells.

Hb D is found in the Punjab and very rarely in UK via the Norfolk regiment some of whom intermarried while stationed in Punjab in the 19th century.

Hb E is found in South-East Asia and is also a mild disease. When these conditions are linked to Hb S or to thalassaemia the condition is more severe.

Haemoglobins which produce methaemoglobinaemia (Hbs M). These are discussed earlier. The patient is not anaemic and is cyanosed. Some patients are polycythaemic because the haemoglobin gives up oxygen less readily than normal haemoglobin. Thus the marrow compensates by increasing red cell production and hence the amount of haemoglobin. There is interference with the normal haem-haem interaction whereby the haem subunits separate to facilitate exchange of oxygen. These high affinity haemoglobins usually but not always (Hb San Diego) have an abnormal electrophoretic mobility and some like Chesapeake and Cape Town are fast moving haemoglobins (anodal to Hb A). The oxygen dissociation curve is shifted to the left with a low P_{50}.

Low-affinity oxygen haemoglobins. Some abnormal haemoglobins give up oxygen more readily than normal. Thus the tissues are able to get enough oxygen even when the haemoglobin concentration is only 8 g/100 ml, e.g. Hb Hammersmith and also Hb S. The patients have a haemolytic anaemia.

Unstable haemoglobins. These patients have a haemolytic anaemia and must be differentiated from other patients with non-spherocytic haemolytic anaemia. They may have Heinz bodies particularly after splenectomy. They have dark urine due to excretion of breakdown product of haem (dipyrroles). The haemoglobin gives an abnormal heat stability test.

The amino acid substitution is such as to interfere with the binding of the haem group within the helix of the globin chain. When the haem is dislodged the chain unfolds and precipitates as a Heinz body. Attacks are often aggravated by drugs such as sulphonamides. The commonest is Hb Koln.

Thalassaemia

These are a group of inherited blood diseases due to failure to make enough α- or β-globin chain of haemoglobin. It is widespread throughout the Mediterranean, Middle East and Asia.

β-thalassaemia major

Both parents (heterozygotes) carry the dominant trait of β-thalassaemia and the patient (homozygote) inherits this from each parent.

There is reduced production of messenger RNA required for β-globin chain synthesis (β+thalassaemia) and in the β° thalassaemia mRNA is entirely absent or is entirely inactive.

The child becomes severely anaemic within the first year of life with an enlarged spleen and liver due to extramedullary blood formation. The X-ray appearance of the bones may be abnormal due to marked haemopoiesis. The skull in particular shows bossing and a 'hair-on end' appearance.

The haemoglobin level will fall to 2–3 g per 100 ml with a markedly hypochromic picture. MCV, MCH and MCHC are low. The blood film shows not only hypochromia but target cells, many bizarre red cell fragments and pyknotic normoblasts. Reticulocyte numbers are never very high despite severe anaemia (usually 4–10 per cent) indicating failure of marrow response.

The bone marrow is active with many red cell precursors. Normoblasts show poor haemoglobinization, irregular pyknotic nuclei and occasionally pale blue staining cytoplasmic inclusions (free α-chains). The latter are better seen on methyl violet staining. There is failure to make enough β-globin chains and hence the excess α-chains accumulate and precipitate in the cell. This is believed to result in the early elimination of these red cells. Most cells fail to complete development in the marrow (ineffective haemopoiesis).

Almost all the haemoglobin is Hb F with the remainder being Hb A_2 which may be either low, normal or slightly raised. Oxygen is not given up as readily from Hb F (the major haemoglobin) as from Hb A and this further impairs tissue oxygenation. There are also small amounts of free α-chains. Some patients have a total absence of Hb A (homozygous β-thalassaemia $\beta°$ type); others have low levels of Hb A.

A few children (about 7 per cent) remain with a haemoglobin level of 6 to 7 g per 100 ml (so called thalassaemia intermedia) but the rest require regular blood transfusions. This leads to a steady accumulation of iron leading to cardiac, endocrine and hepatic damage. Puberty does not occur, there is growth retardation and death in the second decade of life usually from heart failure. In many children the spleen becomes very large and is often removed although the benefits of this step are uncertain.

Many of these consequences can be prevented by iron chelation, (parenteral desferrioxamine) as a subcutaneous infusion with ascorbate over 12 hours each day. This reverses the iron overload and many of the clinical problems accompanying this.

Apart from attempting to prevent marriage of heterozygotes by genetic counselling, antenatal prediction is used. A sample of fetal blood obtained by direct vision is analysed by globin chain synthesis for absence of β-chain formation. Such pregnancies may be terminated. The procedure still carries a significant risk to the fetus however.

β-thalassaemia minor. This very common condition may be suspected from the blood count because the MCV and MCH are low (about 60 fl and 20 pg respectively) but the red cell count is relatively high (above 5·5 million). The haemoglobin level is between 11–12 g/100 ml. The blood film is hypochromic. Confirmation of the diagnosis is made by finding a raised Hb A_2 level (3·5 to 7 per cent). If the Hb A_2 is normal, and the patient does not have iron deficiency, α-thalassemia trait is likely.

Clinically these patients are well and no treatment is required. Genetically they are heterozygotes for β-thalassaemia, that is they have one normal gene and one β-thalassaemia gene.

α-thalassaemia

There are probably two genetic loci controlling α-chain production so that a diploid cell has four genes. In α-thalassaemia one or more genes are absent. The disease may appear as:

1. *Death of the fetus in utero (hydrops fetalis).* In these infants all four α-chain genes are deleted. These infants are oedematous and if not

dead, die within an hour of birth. There is severe anaemia with a thalassaemia-major-type blood picture. Haemoglobin is mainly Hb Barts ($\gamma4$) with small amounts of Hb H ($\beta4$). Both parents are heterozygotes (see 3.)

2. *Haemoglobin H disease*. This is a well defined haemolytic anaemia seen in Greeks and Chinese. Three of 4 α-chain genes are deleted. The haemoglobin levels are between 7–10 g/100 ml with elevated reticulocytes. Haemoglobin H is very unstable. It is made of 4 β chains and this tends to precipitate out of the red cell and appear in the diluting fluid when chamber counts are being made. It may be visualized as stippling in red cells incubated with brilliant cresyl blue. On electrophoresis HbH is one of the fast-moving haemoglobins but the overall amount is often low (less than 20 per cent) because much is lost by precipitation. Hb A_2 is reduced. The new born with Haemoglobin H disease has 20 to 40 per cent Hb Barts in cord blood.

The patients may have an enlarged liver and spleen. The blood film shows microcytosis, target cells and hypochromia with many irregularly crenated red cells. Both parents are heterozygotes (3 and 4 below).

3. *α-thalassaemia trait* (α-Thalassaemia-1). The blood is similar to that described in β-thalassaemia trait with an MCV of the order of 60–70 fl and MCH of 20–24 pg. The Hb A_2 level may be low. Diagnosis may be confirmed by showing depression of α-chain synthesis and hence a low ratio of α/β globin chains of less than one. Occasionally Hb H may be demonstrated in red cells. Two of the α-chain genes are deleted.

4. *Mild α-thalassaemia trait* ('Silent' carrier state or α-Thalassaemia-2). A mild form of α-thalassaemia is common in Indians, Arabs in Saudi-Arabia and West Africans that is not apparently associated with Hb H disease or *hydrops fetalis*. The MCV is often between 68–77 fl and MCH between 21–25 pg. Hb A_2 is generally normal. The red cell count is usually elevated and they have a low α/β globin chain ratio. There is deletion of one of the four α-chain genes.

Thalassaemia in the newborn. The adult or child who cannot make α-chains for the synthesis of Hb A (($\alpha_2\beta_2$) is left with a surplus of β-chains and hence tends to make tetramers like β_4. *In utero* the main haemoglobin is haemoglobin F ($\alpha_2\gamma_2$) and if α-chains cannot be made there is a surplus of γ chains. *In utero* the tetramer is γ_4 (Hb Barts). In hydrops fetalis due to deletion of all α-chain genes, cord blood haemoglobin is almost all Hb Barts and some Hb H.

The newborn with Hb H disease has 25 per cent Hb Barts, and the newborn with α-thalassaemia trait has about 1–5 per cent Hb Barts. Production of both γ-chains and fetal haemoglobin is normally shut off before birth and hence Hb Barts disappears after about three months of age. In the normal newborn the normal MCV is between 95–105 fl and in α-thalassaemia trait it is 80–95 fl. Thus measurement of the MCV (and MCH) in cord blood is a good index of α-thalassaemia in the newborn.

Unusually a defect of α-globin chain synthesis arises from a defect other than gene deletion.

$\delta\beta$-*thalassaemia*. Here there is defective synthesis of both δ- and β-chains. In the homozygous form there is anaemia which is not as severe as in homozygous β-thalassaemia with a haemoglobin level of 9–12 g/100 ml and a microcytic blood picture. The haemoglobin consists of only fetal haemoglobin and a complete absence of Hb A and A$_2$.

Heterozygotes show a blood picture similar to that of β-thalassaemia. The mean haemoglobin level is about 12·5 g/100 ml. Hb A$_2$ is usually normal and Hb F is increased to between 5–15 per cent. In addition the Kleihauer test shows that increased fetal haemoglobin is present in about half the red cells and the remainder staining normally.

Haemoglobin Lepore. The blood is like that in β-thalassaemia trait. Haemoglobin electrophoresis shows a major peak of Hb A, Hb Lepore (6–15 per cent) migrating in a similar position to Hb S and a normal Hb A$_2$. Hb F is slightly raised. Hb Lepore consists of part of the δ-chain and part of the β-chain which have become linked because of a crossing over of chromosomes. The loci for δ- and β-chain genes are normally close together and here it is suggested that there is a fused $\delta\beta$-gene as a result of crossing over of chromosomes.

Hereditary persistence of fetal haemoglobin. In these disorders production of Hb F and hence γ-chains persist into adult life. It is seen in negroes and Greeks. The haemoglobin concentration is normal. The homozygote has a 100 per cent Hb F with no Hb A or Hb A$_2$. The heterozygote has a Hb F concentration of between 15–35 per cent in negroes and the level is somewhat lower in Greek cases.

Haemoglobin Q-α-thalassaemia. This is common in Asia. No α-chains are made. The blood is similar to that seen in Hb H disease with H-inclusion bodies. Haemoglobin electrophoresis shows Hb H, Hb Barts and Hb Q. There is no Hb A.

Haemoglobin Constant Spring-α-thalassaemia. This α-chain variant found on electrophoresis is unusual in that the α-chain in addition to its usual 141 aminoacid residues has an additional 31 residues attached at the end. Clinically the blood picture resembles Hb H disease.

α-thalassaemia-β-thalassaemia combination. This relatively mild disease appears when one parent has α-thalassaemia and the other β-thalassaemia. The α/β-chain ratio is virtually unity and because synthesis of both are equally depressed there is no surplus of either α- or β-chains which in the uncomplicated homozygous β-thalassaemia is responsible for reduced red cell life span.

Other combinations. α- or β-thalassaemia may occur in combination with Hb S, C or E.

Sideroblastic anaemia

A sideroblast is a normoblast stained by Perls's Prussian blue method to show cytoplasmic iron granules. A pathological sideroblast is one in which there is an abnormally large accumulation of iron. Where the iron granules are arranged ring-wise around the nucleus the cell is called a ringed sideroblast (Fig. 13.7). These cells fail to make adequate amounts of haemoglobin (hence the accumulation of iron) and the defect may lie in a failure of haem synthesis. Such a cell may either die in the marrow or if it matures, develop into a hypochromic red cell.

Clinically patients with sideroblastic anaemia complain of the effects of anaemia, *viz*, shortness of breath and lethargy.

The blood picture in a severe case is that of a hypochromic anaemia, but the blood film characteristically shows a mixture of hypochromic and normochromic red cells. Such a dimorphic picture can also arise after iron treatment in iron deficiency, or after transfusion of normal blood to patient with a hypochromic anaemia.

The marrow shows failure of haemoglobinization in one of two ways. Some normoblasts show persistent cytoplasmic basophilia despite maturation of the nucleus. Other normoblasts have an empty cytoplasm with a faint rim of cytoplasm and a pyknotic nucleus. The marrow can be of increased or normal cellularity. Serum iron is generally normal or raised. The disorders associated with pathological sideroblasts are:

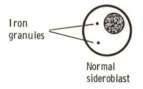

Fig. 13.7 Erythroblasts stained for iron.

1. Marrow toxicity, especially alcohol and drugs like chloramphenicol, and pyridoxine antagonists used in the treatment of tuberculosis such as isoniazid and cycloserine.
2. Congenital sideroblastic anaemia. This is familial occurring in males and transmitted by females.
3. Acquired sideroblastic anaemia. This is generally a refractory anaemia in middle or later life.
4. As part of erythaemic myelosis (Di Guglielmo's disease), a variant of acute leukaemia.

Because of ineffective haemopoiesis there is a high folate requirement and some patients may become folate deficient and megaloblastic. In these some improvement is obtained with folic acid. Others develop a high requirement for pyridoxine and in these a further partial response is obtained with pyridoxine at a dose level of 100–200 mg/day. Those examples due to drugs or alcohol resolve following drug withdrawal.

Dyserythropoietic anaemias. There are a number of rare ill-understood anaemias often seen in childhood. One of these is associated with normoblasts having two or more nuclei in the normoblasts. Occasionally such cases give a positive Ham's test.

References

Dean J, Schechter A N 1978 Sickle-cell anaemia: molecular and cellular basis of therapeutic approaches. New England Journal of Medicine 299: 752–763, 804–811, 863–870
Prankerd T A J, Bellingham A J 1975 Clinics in Haematology, Haemolytic anaemias. Saunders, London
Weatherall D J Clegg J B 1979 The thalassaemia syndromes. Blackwell, Oxford

14

Disorders of platelets

Thrombocytopenias
Idiopathic thrombocytopenic purpura
Drug-induced thrombocytopenic purpura
Thrombocytopenia secondary to other disorders
Qualitative disorders

Platelet disorders are characterized by bleeding and petechial
haemorrhages in skin and mucous membranes. Disorders of platelets
can be due to reduced numbers or to abnormalities of platelet function.
The causes of thrombocytopenia are given in Table 14.1. The
commonest form of thrombocytopenia is idiopathic thrombocytopenic purpura.

Table 14.1 Some causes of thrombocytopenia

Cause	Condition
Decreased production	Marrow aplasia
	Marrow infiltration
	Cytotoxic therapy
Shortened survival	Idiopathic thrombocytopenic purpura
	Drug induced purpura
Increased consumption	Disseminated intravascular coagulation
	Haemangiomas
Sequestration	Hypersplenism
Dilution	Massive transfusion with stored blood

Idiopathic thrombocytopenic purpura (ITP)
Although the common form of 'primary' thrombocytopenic purpura is
called idiopathic, a number of causative factors are known to be
important and it is likely that this is not a uniform entity.

Acute thrombocytopenia is often of acute onset; generalized purpura
appears rapidly in a previously well child or adult. This is the common
form in children, the highest incidence being at about the age of seven.
About half the children have had an infection about 3–6 weeks before
the bleeding appeared. This infection may be a mild upper respiratory
infection, measles, German measles, chicken pox, mumps, cytomegalo
virus or glandular fever. Even vaccination for smallpox or measles has
been followed by purpura. Both sexes are equally affected.

Chronic thrombocytopenia. Chronic thrombocytopenia (Werlhof's disease) may start as an acute disease in childhood or young adults, but more often has an insidious onset with minor bruising and scattered petechiae usually on the legs. Episodes of bleeding may be separated by periods of years during which the platelet count is normal. Others have persistently low platelet counts with little bruising, some having failed to respond to therapy during an acute phase. It is a disorder of adults affecting women more often than men.

During the acute phase purpura appears in all areas of the body and most prominently on the legs. Large bruises follow minor trauma. Women may have severe menstrual bleeding. Haemorrhagic bullae may occur in the mouth. Gastroinestinal haemorrhage and haematuria occur.

Cause. There is considerable evidence that ITP is an autoimmune disease.

There is an association between ITP and other autoimmune disorders such as autoimmune haemolytic anaemia, autoimmune neutropenia, primary biliary cirrhosis and disseminated lupus erythematosus. Like all these disorders, ITP responds to steroid treatment.

Demonstration of platelet antibodies has proved more difficult. New-born infants from women who have ITP may be severely thrombocytopenic and the infant's platelets return to normal after 1–2 months. It is believed that the neonatal thrombocytopenia is due to passage of platelet antibodies across the placenta. Plasma or globulin from patients with ITP when given to subjects with normal platelet counts, causes a sharp fall in platelet levels. Nevertheless more direct attempts at demonstrating humoral platelet antibodies are usually negative. However, most patients can be shown to have an increased amount of IgG coating their platelets using a complement-consumption technique. There is also cell-mediated immunity to platelets using the patients own lymphocytes and their own platelets. Well over half the patients with ITP give positive results with MIF tests (Ch. 7). Whether the virus-related forms of thrombocytopenia are also mediated through an antibody mechanism is not known.

Investigation. Apart from evidence of bleeding and purpura, examination is usually negative. The spleen is generally not palpable. In the uncomplicated case blood shows a low platelet count (generally less than $20 \times 10^9/l$. if the patient has fresh purpura), but the haemoglobin level and white cell count are normal. Occasionally the direct antiglobulin test on the red cells is positive.

ESR is characteristically low, and the blood biochemistry is normal.

The marrow generally shows normal granulopoiesis and erythro-poiesis. There are abundant rounded-up megakaryocytes few of which show platelet budding present on the megakaryocytes of normal marrow. This absence of platelets on megakaryocytes reflects rapid platelet turnover rather than a failure of production.

The commoner disorders that must be differentiated from ITP are acute leukaemia and aplastic anaemia. These are usually easily diagnosed on marrow aspirate or trephine. In patients with thrombocytopenia due to disseminated lupus erythematosus, the ESR is usually high and antinuclear factor and LE cells detected in the blood.

The marrrow is essentially the same in ITP, DLE and drug-induced purpura, and a careful enquiry into drug ingestion is mandatory in all cases. Other less common causes of thrombo-cytopenia are mentioned elsewhere. *Henoch-Schönlein* or *anaphylac-toid purpura*, a common disorder of children, presents with a rash, abdominal pain and joint involvement. The rash however, consists of red macules seen on legs, thighs, and buttocks. It is easily differentiated from ITP by the normal platelet count.

Management. The objective is to restore the platelet count to normal where this is possible. But active therapy is not always indicated. There are various options: no therapy, steroids, immunosuppressive drugs, splenectomy or a combination of these.

Wherever possible therapy should be withheld for up to 10 days in case the diagnosis is a drug-induced purpura. Should this be the case, drug withdrawal alone will restore the platelet count. Children who do not have active bleeding can be left untreated as 97 per cent recover spontaneously, most of them within three months of the onset of the disease. Adults having platelet levels between 30 to $80 \times 10^9/l.$ and only occasional bruising also need not be given active treatment. The platelet levels tend to fluctuate and in many become normal without treatment. These are probably examples of chronic ITP.

In practice children or adults with active bleeding will require treatment which should be steroids in the first instance. Prednisone (40–80 mg/day) is adequate and is usually associated with a rise in platelets within a few days. Whether steroids suppress antibody formation, suppress phagocytosis of antibody-coated platelets by macrophages, or non-specifically decrease capillary fragility, is uncertain. Those who respond should be kept on steroids for two to four weeks after the platelet count is normal and then steroids are tailed off over another 4–8 weeks. Children and young adults who continue to have fresh bleeding after four weeks of steroid therapy should undergo splenectomy. Each patient obviously requires independent assessment Some may show a small rise in platelet levels with only minor bruising and in these steroids should be continued up to 10–12 weeks before considering steroid therapy to have failed.

Older patients who fail to respond to steroids should be treated with immunosuppressive drugs. This is not desirable in young patients since some like cyclophosphamide, may cause sterility by damaging germ cells. Vincristine (1–2 mg i.v. every 7 to 10 days) for not less than three doses, cyclophosphamide (100 mg/day) or azathioprine (100 mg/day) have all proved successful and smaller maintenance doses of the latter two may be required. If there is no response after six weeks it should be regarded as a failure. Patients who continue to bleed despite prednisone and immunosuppressive drugs should undergo splenectomy.

Splenectomy removes the major organ responsible for platelet destruction. In a successful splenectomy the platelets may rise within 1–2 days of the operation, sometimes only after 7–10 days. Not all patients respond to splenectomy. One quarter will remain with reduced platelet levels although few will have purpura. Relapse after splenectomy must be treated with prednisone and immunosuppressive drugs and there is a greater likelihood of success after the operation. Platelet transfusions are of little value since the platelets disappear from the circulation within 1–2 hours of infusion. They may be of more use if given at the time of splenectomy. Nevertheless, it may be necessary to give platelets in the presence of severe bleeding, for example gastrointestinal or intracranial.

The natural history of chronic ITP is that of a disease that undergoes spontaneous remissions and relapses over many years.

Drug-induced thrombocytopenic purpura

Clinically these patients present in the same way as patients with acute ITP. They may be taking a variety of drugs or may not admit that they are taking any at all. Withdrawal of the drug should produce a remission within 1–2 weeks.

Some drugs like the thiazide diuretics or cytotoxic drugs may act directly on megakaryocytes. Others act through immunological mechanisms which are the same as those described in relation to drug-induced haemolytic anaemia (Ch. 13). A large number of drugs are occasionally associated with immune thrombocytopenia including paracetamol, aspirin, phenylbutazone, sulphonamides, quinine and quinidine, sedormid, diphenylhydantoin, barbiturates, tolbutamide, digoxin, gold, etc.

Laboratory demonstration of drug-sensitization affecting platelets is usually unsatisfactory. It is claimed that complement-fixation and antiglobulin consumption tests using platelets, the drug and patients serum, and tests involving the release of platelet factor 3 or platelet aggregation, are the most satisfactory. Older tests which involve clot retraction which occurred in the absence of the drug and was inhibited in its presence, are insensitive, but very helpful if demonstrated.

Occasionally when it is necessary to give the patient the drug therapeutically, clinical challenge may be necessary using a very small single dose of the drug (in μg rather the mg quantities) and following the platelet level hourly. There may be a very abrupt fall in platelet levels but sometimes this only occurs with a larger dose. Thus re-introduction of a possible offending drug must be done with caution. Thrombocytopenia due to gold injections given in rheumatoid arthritis may persist until the gold has been removed by giving injections of BAL (British anti-lewisite).

Thrombocytopenia secondary to other disorders

Decreased production of platelets in the bone marrow occurs in marrow aplasia, in leukaemia, megaloblastic anaemia, after treatment with cytotoxic drugs, or if marrow is replaced by malignant tissue. *Increased* consumption is the cause of thrombocytopenia in giant haemangiomata of children and in disseminated intravascular coagulation. A combination of splenic *sequestration*, consumption and decreased production, contribute to the thrombocytopenia of chronic liver disease.

Blood transfusions exceeding 10 units may result in a fall in platelet count due to dilution, but rarely in bleeding unless associated with loss of other coagulation factors. By-pass surgery with an extracorporeal circulation regularly results in marked falls in platelet numbers. These recover several days after surgery. Inadequate neutralization of heparin and DIC are the more usual causes of bleeding in these patients.

Thrombotic thrombocytopenic purpura is a rare, acute and usually rapidly fatal disorder characterized by a haemolytic anaemia, renal damage, bleeding and neurological abnormalities. The cause is not known. There is widespread occlusion of small vessels due to small thrombi consisting of platelet aggregates. The patient may present with purpura, jaundice, anaemia and fever. The blood shows a low haemoglobin level, reticulocytosis, low platelet count and leucocytosis. The blood film shows red cell fragments. Coagulation tests give very variable results and some patients show evidence of DIC. The majority of patients die. Treatment is with steroids in large doses; plasma exchange, fresh frozen plasma and antiplatelet drugs are also used. Individual circumstances may suggest splenectomy or heparin if there is evidence of continuing DIC.

Post-transfusion purpura. Severe thrombocytopenia may appear about one week after a blood transfusion and may persist for 3–7 weeks. All the eight cases reported hitherto have been in women who have had children. A platelet antibody appears in these patients against a platelet antigen Zw or Pl^{A1}. This antigen is present in 98 per cent of persons but is lacking in these patients. This would suggest that there is an immunological basis to this thrombocytopenia similar to that in a delayed transfusion reaction. The marrow is similar to that in ITP.

Qualitative disorders of platelets

This is a group of disorders characterized by a bleeding diathesis due to an abnormality in platelet function. Amongst these disorders are:

Congenital
1. Glanzmann's thrombasthenia.
2. Bernard-Soulier syndrome.
3. Inherited defects of the release reaction.

Acquired
1. Drug induced.
2. Part of a myeloproliferative disorder.
3. Renal disease.

Patients suffering from congenital disorders have a life-long history of bleeding from skin and mucous membranes, easy bruising, menorrhagia, and sometimes excessive blood loss at surgery. Family history is often positive. Typical laboratory and diagnostic features are presented in Table 14.2. As von Willebrand's syndrome and aspirin ingestion are the most common diagnostic alternatives, they are also included in the Table.

Thrombasthenia is due to deficiency of a platelet membrane glycoprotein. Such platelets fail to aggregate to ADP, collagen, thrombin and ristocetin. It is an autosomal recessive disorder, resulting in a moderately severe haemorrhagic tendency.

Bernard-Soulier syndrome is an autosomal recessive defect of platelet adhesion to subendothelium. The patients have a variably reduced platelet count, defective prothrombin consumption and many giant platelets on the blood film. The platelets aggregate normally to ADP, collagen and thrombin, but fail to aggregate to ristocetin or bovine fibrinogen.

Defects of the platelet release reaction are found in many clinical

Table 14.2 Results of tests in disorders of platelet function

Disease	Mode of inheritance	Platelet count	Platelet morphology	Retention on glass beads	ADP	Aggregation Adrenaline	Collagen	Ristocetin
Thrombasthenia	Autosomal recessive	Normal	Normal	Reduced	Absent	Absent	Absent	Absent
Bernard Soulier syndrome	?Autosomal recessive	Low	Giant forms	Reduced	Normal	Normal	Normal	Absent
Defects of platelet release	?	Normal	Normal	Normal	Absent secondary wave	Absent	Absent	Normal or absent
Aspirin ingestion	–	Normal	Normal	Normal	Absent secondary wave	Absent	Absent	Normal or absent
von Willebrand's syndrome	Autosomal dominant	Normal	Normal	Reduced or normal	Normal	Normal	Normal	Absent

conditions; the platelets do not aggregate on exposure to collagen and disaggregate after the addition of ADP. The hereditary disorders of the release reaction can be divided into those due to storage pool deficiency (failure of release is due to a lack of normal storage sites for ADP), those due to an abnormality of the release mechanism in the presence of a normal storage pool, and those due to a defect of nucleotide synthesis secondary to chronic hypoglycaemia, as in glycogen storage disease, type I. Similar acquired disorder of the release reaction may be found in myelo-proliferative disorders, renal disease, intravascular coagulation and after taking aspirin or other non-steroidal anti-inflammatory drugs.

It is occasionally necessary to distinguish between von Willebrand's syndrome and other forms of platelet dysfunction. In von Willebrand's syndrome platelets aggregate normally to ADP, adrenaline and collagen, but fail to aggregate to ristocetin. It is sometimes possible to demonstrate impaired retention in glass bead columns and the levels of factor VIII clotting activity and antigen are reduced.

In most cases the bleeding tendency is mild and no treatment is required. Platelet transfusions may be necessary in severely affected patients requiring surgery. Menorrhagia is troublesome in many women and may be controlled with the contraceptive pill. The patients should be advised never to take aspirin or anti-inflammatory drugs which may aggravate the bleeding tendency.

References
Hardisty R M 1978 Disorders of platelet function. British Medical Bulletin 33: 207–212
Wintrobe M M 1975 Clinical Haematology. Lee & Febiger, Philadelphia p. 1071–1118

15

Disorders affecting all the blood elements

Marrow failure	*Myeloproliferative disorders*
Aplastic anaemia	Polycythaemia rubra vera
Transient marrow failure	chronic myelofibrosis
Pure red cell aplasia;	Familial polycythaemia

Aplastic and hypoplastic anaemia

When the marrow fails to produce adequate numbers of cells the patient becomes anaemic, has a low white cell count (leucopenia) and a low platelet count (thrombocytopenia). The term pancytopenia describes depression of all these cells in the peripheral blood.

Causative factors

Drugs. Many chemical substances can depress the marrow and occasionally produce irreversible damage. Many of these chemicals are used in treatment of diseases and others are used in industry. The vast majority of persons taking these drugs or exposed to these chemicals, are unaffected; the rare patient proves susceptible. As an example over a three year period in the United Kingdom about 10 million prescriptions were issued for the anti-rheumatic drug, phenyl-butazone. During this period some 139 cases of aplastic anaemia were reported associated with the use of this drug, of which 101 proved fatal. In the UK a register of adverse drug reactions is maintained by the Committee of Safety of Medicines. If any drug is suspected of having been responsible for marrow damage the register can be consulted to see if such reactions have been noted in relation to administration of the drug in the past. It is not known why a small minority of patients are susceptible to marrow damage by a drug that is well tolerated by the vast majority.

Drugs that are associated with aplastic anaemia are phenylbutazone and oxyphenylbutazone, chloramphenical, aspirin (acetylsalicylic acid) penicillin, sulphonamides, gold-compounds, and many others. Chemical substances include benzene, arsenicals, DDT and others.

Other drugs are used in treatment of malignant disease and over-dosage may lead to transient, more rarely to irreversible aplasia. These are alkylating, agents (chlorambucil, cyclophosphamide, melphalan, busulphan), procarbazine, methotrexate, fluorouracil and others. A very careful history must be taken from the patient about exposure to drugs or chemicals both at home and at work.

Radiation. Exposure to irradiation may lead to aplastic anaemia, loss of lymphocytes being followed by neutropenia and reticulocytopenia and finally by thrombocytopenia. Inadequate protection of radiologists in the past has led to aplasia.

Congenital. (Fanconi's anaemia). This is a form of aplastic anaemia found in children generally after the age of 4. It is usually associated with congenital abnormalities (short stature, squint, small head—microcephaly—and additional thumb). Patients also have a raised fetal haemoglobin level, a variety of chromosomal abnormalities and often a family history of the disease.

Autoimmune. The development of methods for culture of haemopoietic stem cells has revealed factors in the blood from some patients with aplastic anaemia that inhibited development of colonies. In some cases these have been humoral factors and required complement and in others it has been due to T-lymphoid cell activity.

Virus-induced. Aplasia may follow infectious hepatitis. Whether other viruses have a similar action is not known.

Idiopathic. In about half the cases an adequate cause is not found.

Clinical aspects

Patients complain of lethargy and weakness due to anaemia, of a tendency to bruise with undue ease due to loss of platelets, and less frequently, of an inability to overcome infections because of neutropenia. It may occur at any age and in either sex. In some the illness usually bleeding, may develop abruptly.

Examination shows pallor, purpura and less frequently, signs of infection. Nowadays, some patients come to light because of unexplained macrocytosis in the blood count and this can precede significant anaemia by many months.

Investigation

Blood count shows anaemia, leucopenia and thrombocytopenia. Often one or two cell lines are depressed to a more significant extent than others. Thus the patient with a bleeding tendency may have about 8·0 g of haemoglobin/100 ml with a white cell count of about 1800 cells/μl and platelets of only 10 000/μl. There are no abnormal cells in the film. Macrocytosis is almost the rule and in some the MCV may be as high as in severe megaloblastic anaemia. Surprisingly reticulocytes are often at the 2–3 per cent level and it has been suggested that there is delayed maturation into mature erythrocytes.

Marrow may be difficult to aspirate and repeated attempts may be required. Typically the marrow shows fat, some lymphocytes, iron-storage-type reticulum cells and only few haemopoietic cells. There are various pitfalls. It may prove impossible to aspirate adequate marrow. Even when marrow aspiration is impossible, fluid from the marrow needle will generally provide confirmation of one of the alternate diagnoses which is leukaemia. A marrow trephine is essential in all cases to confirm marrow aplasia.

Not uncommonly, foci of surviving haemopoietic tissue persist in the marrow and aspiration from such a site provides the contrast of pancytopenia in the peripheral blood with apparently normal marrow. Once again a marrow trephine is necessary as well as aspiration of marrow from another site. Old people often have fatty hypocellular marrows which must not be mistaken for hypoplastic anaemia. Finally, radiotherapy for cancer of the breast or for a tumour of the lung even if carried out many years previously, will destroy haemopoiesis in the sternum permanently and aspiration from this site will show total aplasia.

Other studies. The marrow can be visualized with a gamma camera after an injection of a very shortlived isotope of iron (^{52}Fe), and where available, confirms absence of erythropoiesis.

The serum iron level is abnormally high with saturation of transferrin. Occasionally a positive result is obtained with Ham's test (for PNH). Erythropoietin levels are elevated. Coagulation tests reflect the low platelet count (prolonged bleeding time, positive Hess test and poor clot retraction).

Iron-kinetic studies are often useful in diagnosis of a difficult case. The plasma iron clearance is abnormally slow indicating poor uptake of iron by the marrow and there is a very low incorporation of the labelled iron into red cells over the next two weeks.

The two common disorders that must be differentiated from marrow failure are acute leukaemia and thrombocytopenic purpura.

Management
This consists of:

1. Search and elimination of possible drug or chemical cause.
2. Supportive therapy.
3. Restoration of marrow function.
4. Marrow transplantation.

Supportive therapy consists of blood and platelet transfusions when required. When the patient is first seen blood should be collected for genotyping and determination of HLA group. Some patients may require regular transfusions and hence may thereafter always have a mixture of transfused as well as their own red cells. Knowledge of the patients own red cell antigens may simplify solution of future cross-matching problems. Antibiotics are given when required. Severe neutropenia with infection may on occasion justify isolation procedures.

Patients with severe bruising, severe anaemia and a very low white cell count are likely to do badly and die within months or weeks. Most adults do not do well with a mortality of about 70 per cent. Children tend to do rather better. Spontaneous remissions occur even as long as after two years. Other patients stabilize with moderate anaemia and a reduced platelet count.

Androgens may stimulate marrow recovery. Oxymethalone (up to 300 mg/day is used) but others may be better. The effect may not be evident until three months have elapsed and it should not be abandoned before this length of time. However, in recent years the efficacy of androgens has been questioned and it is true that a properly controlled clinical trial has not been performed.

Toxic effects of androgens are their virilizing action (hirsutism, acne, change of voice and sometimes increased libido). They may produce a cholestatic jaundice. This may be detected biochemically by an increase in plasma transaminase and bilirubin levels and by clinical jaundice. The jaundice is reversed by withdrawal of therapy. Some elevation of transaminase levels may be an indication to reduce the dose of androgens but not necessarily to withdraw treatment.

Steroids are of doubtful value but should be given if there is no evidence of response to androgens after three months or if purpura is persistent. Some of those who respond to androgens may require a smaller maintenance dose. Success has been claimed with administration of antithymocyte globulin and antilymphocyte globulin but controlled trials have not been performed.

Some 50 per cent of patients with aplastic anaemia who have received a marrow transplant from a HLA identical donor, usually a sibling, have had a successful outcome many with a long survival. The conditions for success are a transplant within the first 3 months of the illness and before many blood transfusions have been given. The best results are in those under 21 years of age. The immediate complications are graft rejection, graft versus host disease and severe infections. The treatment has been used for the most severely affected patients.

Transient marrow failure

Marrow failure that may occur in the course of a chronic haemolytic anaemia and associated with minor infections has been discussed in Chapter 13.

Some of the drugs that may result in aplastic anaemia can produce toxic but reversible marrow changes that lead to a pancytopenia lasting several days after the drugs are withdrawn. Thus chloramphenical at a dose of 2 g/day regularly produces marrow changes. Alcoholic intoxication also has this effect. In the marrow these changes are ringed sideroblasts, vacuolation in all types of marrow cells and megaloblastic changes in erythroblasts. Drug withdrawal results in reversal of these changes but at least in the case of chloramphenicol, continuation of the drug may lead to permanent damage.

Pure red cell aplasia

Congenital. This is a severe form of anaemia seen within the first few months of life. White cells and platelets are normal. The red cells may be normal in appearance in some cases, but show variable changes in others. Marrow shows normal granulopoiesis and normal megakaryocytes but erythroblasts may be either scanty or show dyshaemopoiesis with binucleate forms. This rare disorder is likely to comprise a number of different biochemical and/or genetic defects including that termed the Diamond-Backfan syndrome. Treatment is by transfusion. Androgens and steroids may be helpful and splenectomy may sometimes help in those failing to respond.

Acquired red cell aplasia

Pure red cell aplasia is a rare disorder of adult life, women being involved twice as often as men. Severe anaemia is present while the white cells and platelets remain entirely normal. About half the patients have a tumour of the thymus gland (thymoma). The thymoma may precede the anaemia by years, coincide with the anaemia or develop some years later. Removal of the thymoma does not necessarily influence the course of the anaemia.

The blood shows macrocytosis, reticulocyte levels are very low or even zero, and the marrow either shows a few degenerate erythroblasts or is entirely devoid of them. Sera from twenty per cent of cases give a positive result in a test for anti-nuclear factor.

The cause seems to be an immunological rejection of erythroblasts, that is, it is an autoimmune disease. The patient's serum prevents haem synthesis in suspension of normal erythoblasts and causes release of ^{59}Fe from normal erythroblasts first incubated with radio-iron.

The outlook is poor and most patients die within a few years of diagnosis. Nevertheless many do respond to steroids or androgens, or to immunosuppressive drugs such as cyclophosphamide. When a thymoma is present it should be removed since half these tumours are malignant. Transfusions are given when needed.

The myeloproliferative disorders

Polycythaemia and chronic myeloid leukaemia represent overproduction of red blood cells and white blood cells respectively. Polycythaemia may evolve into a third disorder called chronic myelofibrosis or may transform into chronic myeloid leukaemia. All three conditions, polycythaemia, chronic granulocytic leukaemia and chronic myelofibrosis may terminate as acute myeloblastic leukaemia. Not uncommonly patients are seen who show features of more than one of these disorders. Because of these relationships, these conditions are grouped as the myeloproliferative disorders (Fig. 15.1). At least two of these disorders, polycythaemia and chronic myeloid leukaemia, are of clonal origin, that is, they arise from a mutation of a single stem cell.

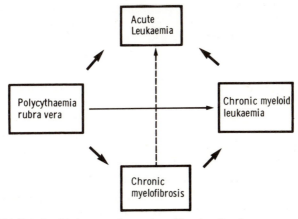

Fig. 15.1 Relationship between the myeloproliferative disorders.

Polycythaemia rubra vera

Here there is excessive marrow production of all the blood elements.

Clinical aspects

It is a disorder of older people. Patients have a high colour (plethora).

They seek medical attention because of headaches, dizziness, visual disturbances, generalized itching aggravated by bathing or thrombotic episodes of leg veins (phlebitis) or of arteries in legs, heart or brain giving rise to intermittent claudication, myocardial infarction, or hemiplegia respectively. There may be haemorrhagic episodes such as large subcutaneous bleeds or bleeding from a peptic ulcer. About one third of patients have a high blood pressure.

Examination often shows an enlarged spleen but if the spleen is more than 10 cm below the costal margin development of myelofibrosis should be suspected.

Blood. The haemoglobin level varies from 18-24 g/100 ml with corresponding increases in the red cell count and PCV. The red cell size is generally normal but sometimes the picture is complicated by iron-deficiency anaemia when the MCV and MCH are reduced. In three quarters of patients the total white cell count is increased to between 12000 to 25000/μl, and in half the patients the platelet count is increased, the range being 450000 to over one million/μl. However, one in five patients has normal platelet and white cell count.

Blood volume. In polycythaemia the total blood volume is increased above the normal range (Ch. 2) by virtue of an increase in the red cell mass. A similar increase in the red cell mass occurs in *secondary polycythaemia* where it is a compensation for failure of normal oxygenation of the blood as in pulmonary disease (e.g. emphysema) or congenital heart disease. Rarely a high-affinity haemoglobin (Ch. 13) or erythropoietin-producing tumours including fibroids in the uterus, hepatoma or some brain tumours may give rise to polycythaemia. Generally these disorders are accompanied by normal white cell and platelet levels.

A high haemoglobin and a high red cell count may also occur in *polycythaemia of stress* (relative polycythaemia). Despite a very high haemoglobin concentration the red cell volume is normal but the plasma volume is markedly reduced, giving haemoconcentration. Some of these patients have a marked anxiety neurosis.

The erythropoietin level is normal or raised in the secondary polycythaemias but immeasurably low in polycythaemia rubra vera.

Essential thrombocythaemia. In some patients the platelet count may be exceptionally high reaching several millions/μl. These patients tend to bleed easily and are often iron deficient and hence the haemoglobin concentration tends to be lower than expected. Such cases are sometimes called essential thrombocythaemia. These must be differentiated from other diseases with high platelet counts such as chronic myelofibrosis, chronic myeloid leukaemia and loss of spleen after surgery (post-splenectomy) or due to splenic atrophy. Occasionally a high platelet count is seen in the absence of these diseases and with a normal white cell count and red cell mass. Platelets in polycythaemia are often functionally abnormal.

Marrow. The marrow shows an increase in cellularity, often low or absent iron stores, but is otherwise unremarkable.

Other findings. Blood uric acid is raised in about $\frac{2}{3}$ of patients. The serum vitamin B_{12} level may be abnormally high due to an increased level of transcobalamin I in plasma and finally the white blood cell alkaline phosphatase score may be raised.

Diagnosis. The diagnosis of polycythaemia rubra vera requires:

1. Confirmation of polycythaemia by showing increases in red cell and total blood volume. If these are equivocal, it is best to repeat the estimation in a few months.
2. If the red cell mass is increased secondary polycythaemia is excluded by:

   a. demonstrating normal oxygen saturation of arterial blood.
   b. demonstrating normal affinity of haemoglobin for oxygen by showing a normal P_{50} (Ch. 3) in a venous blood sample.
   c. demonstrating a virtual absence of erythropoietin from plasma or urine.

Cause. The cause of primary polycythaemia is not known.

Management

Treatment is designed to reduce the red cell volume to within or near normal levels and to reduce the platelet count to normal. This in turn, significantly reduces the risk of thrombotic and other complications of the disease and generally alleviates such symptoms as skin irritation.

Venesection. A series of venesections over a few weeks produce a rapid fall in red cell volume. It is useful in producing rapid relief from headaches and is particularly indicated in patients who have had recent minor transient strokes as such symptoms often precede a major cerebral catastrophe. It is useful in young patients in whom one is more reluctant to give radiation. Venesection however, replaces polycythaemia by iron deficiency and does not deal with the elevated platelet levels.

Chemotherapy. Marrow depressants such as busulphan, chlorambucil and cyclophosphamide can damp down marrow production. Doses are busulphan 4–6 mg daily, chlorambucil 6 mg daily and cyclophosphamide 100 mg daily, and these doses are reduced if maintenance is required. Many months of treatment are needed with regular blood checks. These measures are generally combined with venesections.

Radiotherapy. This is given as radioactive phosphorous (^{32}P). ^{32}P has a half-life of 14·3 days. It is generally incorporated into phosphates and phospholipids throughout the body, about 90 per cent being found in marrow, liver and spleen. Following adminstration of about 5mCi there is some urinary excretion in the next 24 hours. The effects on the blood are seen over about 12 weeks with a fall in white cells and platelets during the first four weeks and a slower decline of red cells over 12 weeks, (Fig. 15.2). Remission may last two years or longer and further doses are given when needed. This treatment requires relatively few follow up visits to the clinician.

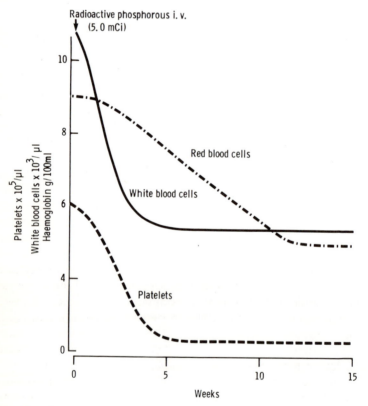

Fig. 15.2 The response of the blood following an injection of radioactive phosphorus.

Associated therapy. Allopurinol may be needed if the uric acid level is elevated to avoid an attack of gout. Hypertension may require treatment. Very intractable pruritus can be controlled with oral cholestyramine.

Prognosis

The median survival after appearance of symptoms is about 13 years. Many die from the thrombotic complications of the disease. About 12 per cent of the patients with polycythaemia appear to develop chronic myelofibrosis and about 10 per cent die of leukaemia, generally acute myeloblastic. In some leukaemia appears as a further complication of myelofibrosis. A multicentre study in which the results of venesection, chlorambucil and radiophosphorus were compared, has been carried out. The best results were in the group receiving ^{32}P. The highest frequency of leukaemia and other neoplasms occured in those given chlorambucil and was attributed to its effect in producing chromosome breaks. The highest incidence of thrombotic complications occurred in those treated only with phlebotomy.

Chronic myelofibrosis

The classical presentation of this disease is of an older patient with a very large spleen. The blood picture is very characteristic. The haemoglobin may be normal, elevated or low. The white count is increased (usually 15–30 000) and platelet count is often elevated. The stained film shows many red cells that are teardrop in shape. There are normoblasts and myelocytes and typically a significant number of myeloblasts. Platelets are abundant. Finally, attempts at marrow aspiration fail to yield material—a so called dry tap.

In this disease excess fibrous tissue is laid down throughout the marrow. This is first detectable in marrow sections by an increased reticulin pattern with silver stains. This is followed by deposition of collagen and in the very late stages by deposition of calcium (myelosclerosis). At the same time the spleen enlarges, not as a compensation for loss of marrow, but as part of the disease process. Extramedullary haemopoiesis is the rule in this disease.

Clinical aspects

The patient may have had long standing polycythaemia. More often they complain of loss of energy due to moderate anaemia, sometimes to pain from a splenic infarct, of discomfort due to an enlarged spleen or to thrombotic complications such as thrombosis in leg veins. In addition, pruritus may be as prominent as is in polycythaemia. Pain can be due to pressure of the spleen on structures passing into the pelvis.

Examination may show a plethoric subject with protuberant abdomen. The spleen is large and may be massive. Liver is often enlarged and liver biopsy may show cirrhosis as well as extramedullary haemopoiesis including sometimes megakaryocytes in the portal tracts, a finding almost diagnostic of myelofibrosis.

Investigation

Diagnosis can be suspected from the appearance of the blood film and must be confirmed by demonstrating increased reticulin/collagen on marrow obtained by trephine biopsy. On occasion it is still possible to aspirate some marrow from particular sites and generally fluid from the marrow needle may provide enough material to check on the nature of haemopoiesis. Generally however, a dry tap results.

Anaemia is often due to marked pooling of blood in the spleen. This is assessed by re-injecting the patients own cells labelled with ^{51}Cr and collecting blood samples at 3, 10, 30 and 60 minutes as in a blood volume estimation. At three minutes the labelled red cells have equilibrated within the circulation outside the spleen and after 30 minutes the red cells have equilibrated with all the red cells including those in the spleen. The difference between red cell volume estimates at 3 and 30 (or 60 minutes) represents the blood in the spleen.

The spleen may also be an important and sometimes the major site for haemopoiesis. This is revealed by giving ^{59}Fe-linked to transferrin. Surface counting shows that instead of the iron clearing to the marrow (sacral counts) it clears to the spleen. Thereafter it slowly leaves the spleen to be incorporated into new red cells.

Plasma uric acid may be elevated, the serum vitamin B_{12} level may be very high due to a high transcobalamin I level and unlike uncomplicated polycythaemia, there is usually evidence of folic-acid deficiency. Serum and red folate levels are often abnormally low. The reason for this is thought to be ineffective haemopoiesis with a relatively high folate requirement. Leucocyte alkaline phosphatase is high by contrast with chronic myeloid leukaemia where it is low.

Management. This is designed to keep the patient comfortable, to prevent thrombotic complications and maintain folate status.

It is often desirable to reduce the size of the spleen because

1. The pool of blood in the spleen results in 'anaemia' and hence considerable lethargy.

2. Splenic infarcts produce both acute as well as chronic nagging pain.
3. The mass of the large spleen is uncomfortable and may make it impossible for patients to bend in order to reach their feet.
4. The spleen may produce pressure on pelvic nerves causing pain.
5. Rarely the spleen is hyperactive and actively destroys red cells, platelets and/or neutrophils (hypersplenism).

Busulphan (4 mg/day) is usually very effective in shrinking the largest spleens with marked clinical benefit and significant rise in haemoglobin concentration. Radiotherapy to the lower end of the spleen may relieve pressure symptoms. Recently there has been a trend to early splenectomy after successful busulphan treatment. There is no published data on whether this is advantageous in the long term. In the short term it can lead to elevated platelet levels and aggravate thrombotic problems. The spleen must never be removed when it is an important site of haemopoiesis.

Thrombotic complications are best dealt with by reducing platelet levels with drugs such as busulphan but some patients may require anti-coagulant therapy.

All patients should be given folic acid five mg daily. Folate deficiency may be suspected by the development of a transfusion requirement and an unexpected fall in the platelet count, both indicating marrow failure. In such cases megaloblasts may be seen in peripheral blood films or buffy coat preparations and even in the fluid obtained from the needle after an apparently failed attempt to aspirate marrow.

Gout is treated with allopurinol.

Ultimately patients die of acute leukaemia, marrow failure or thrombotic complications including myocardial infarction and pulmonary embolism.

Familial polycythaemia

The least rare in this group of disorders is polycythaemia due to abnormal haemoglobins with a high affinity for oxygen so that the P_{50} value is less than normal. The haemoglobin is usually abnormal on electrophoresis but may be normal, for example, in Hb San Diego. The patients are well and have an erythrocytosis which is a compensation for the reluctance of the red cell to give up its oxygen.

References

Glass J L, Wasserman L R 1977 Primary polycythaemia, 2nd edn. In: Williams W J, Beutler E, Erslev A J, Rundles R W (eds) Hematology. McGraw-Hill, New York

Thomas E D 1978 Clinics in haematology. Aplastic anaemia. Saunders, London

16

Congenital abnormalities of blood coagulation

Congenital abnormalities of coagulation are rare. The most common are the defects of factor VIII (haemophilia and von Willebrand's syndrome) and factor IX (haemophilia B or Christmas disease). All are characterized by bleeding from injuries, by epistaxis, menorrhagia, haematuria or gastrointestinal haemorrhage. There may be prolonged bleeding after tooth extraction, after operations, or there may be painful bleeding into joints and bleeding into deep tissue.

Features in the history which favour a coagulation disorder are a long history, haemorrhage affecting different parts of the body and a similar abnormality in one or more relatives. The extent of bleeding after tooth extraction or minor operation is very helpful. Normal people may ooze from a tooth socket for up to 24 hours, but bleeding persisting for more than 24 hours in the absence of infection is probably abnormal particularly if blood transfusion is required. Patients who have undergone major surgery or tonsillectomy without undue haemorrhage are probably not suffering from a congenital haemorrhagic defect.

The family history is important and a family tree should be drawn; the possibility of consanguinity must be explored as many coagulation disorders are inherited as autosomal incompletely recessive characteristics.

Abnormalities of factor VIII—Classical haemophilia

Inheritance. Classical haemophilia is a deficiency of factor VIII clotting activity inherited as a sex-linked recessive disorder (Fig. 16.1).

The genes that code for factor VIII clotting activity are located on the X chromosome. As a rule only males are affected. Females that carry one abnormal gene show levels of factor VIII in plasma that are intermediate between those in normal subjects and haemophiliacs and sometimes have a mild bleeding tendency. The sons of haemophiliacs are normal, but all daughters are carriers. Sons of female carriers of

haemophilia have a 50 per cent chance of having the disease and
daughters have a 50 per cent chance of being carriers. Women
occasionally have low factor VIII levels and some causes for this are
shown in Table 16.1.

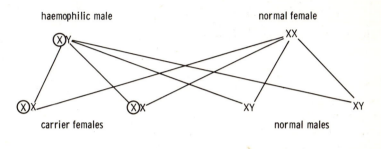

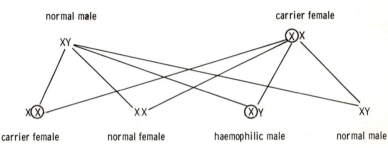

Fig. 16.1 Inheritance of haemophilia A.

Table 16.1   Causes of low factor VIII in women.

1. von Willebrand's syndrome
2. Homozygous female (mother carrier, father haemophiliac)
3. Carrier female with one X chromosome; testicular feminization (46,XY), Turner's
   syndrome (45,XO), mosaicism (46,XX/XO)
4. Extreme lyonization in a carrier female
5. Deletion or translocation involving X chromosome

Between 30 and 40 per cent of patients with haemophilia do not
have a family history and some of them are due to a fresh mutation.

Factor VIIIRAg in haemophilia. When haemophilic plasmas are
allowed to react with antisera against pure factor VIII, prepared in
rabbits, it can be shown that all haemophilic plasmas have factor
VIIIRAg even if no factor VIIIC is demonstrated in conventional
coagulation assays.

Identification of carriers. The identification of carriers is important
in haemophilic families. Possible carriers are sisters of haemophiliacs,
daughters of obligatory carriers (obligatory carriers are daughters of a

haemophiliac), granddaughters of obligatory carriers who have a one in four chance of being carriers and so on. On genetic grounds carrier females are expected to have half the normal plasma factor VIIIC, that is about 50iu/dl. In practice many carriers have normal or even high factor VIIIC levels because plasma factor VIII rises under stress. In addition, many normal individuals have factor VIII levels around 50iu/dl. It is thus possible to identify only about one third of carriers by low factor VIIIC levels. It is helpful to compare the factor VIIIC levels in the possible carrier with those in her healthy brothers and to determine the levels of factor VIIIRAg. If a great excess of factor VIIIRAg is present it is likely that the individual is a carrier of haemophilia.

Manifestations. Patients with haemophilia have levels of factor VIIIC in plasma varying from 0iu/dl to 40iu/dl. The unit is based on the activity of one ml of average fresh normal plasma. The severity of bleeding generally parallels the level of factor VIIIC in plasma (Table 16.2). The severity of haemophilia in any one family tends to remain the same from generation to generation.

Table 16.2   Severity of bleeding and the level of Factor VIIIC

Blood level of factor VIIIC iu/dl	Bleeding
25–40	After major trauma only
5–25	After operations and after minor trauma
1– 5	After minor trauma; occasional spontaneous haemorrhages
0	Spontaneous bleeding into muscles and joints with crippling

Bleeding usually starts at the end of the first year when the child becomes mobile. It affects joints such as knees, ankles, later elbows and shoulders, often in the absence of any obvious injury. These joint bleeds (haemarthroses) are painful and if not treated lead to permanent joint deformity. Bleeding into muscles may cause damage to nerves and arteries, and lead to fibrosis and contractures. A complication of deep tissue bleeding is the formation of large blood cysts (pseudotumours) which gradually erode bone and destroy soft tissues often in the region of the hip. Gastrointestinal bleeding, and painless haematuria are common. Clot formation in the renal pelvis may cause obstruction of urinary flow, and ureteric colic.

Haemophilic patients bleed after any injury or any form of surgery, including dental extraction. Initially there may be no bleeding but after an interval bleeding starts and then, in the absence of effective treatment, may continue for many days and weeks. Bleeding may be more severe for several months, followed by a period when little or no bleeding occurs. As the patient grows older and perhaps becomes more cautious, bleeding episodes become less frequent.

Diagnosis. This is suggested by the history and confirmed by laboratory tests. Typical findings are shown in Table 16.3. In severe or moderately severe haemophilia, the laboratory findings are characteristic. In mildly affected patients the screening tests may be normal and assays are needed for diagnosis.

Table 16.3   Coagulation tests in haemophilia

Test	Normal	Haemophilia		
		Mild	Moderate	Severe
Whole blood clotting time, min	2–7	5	10	>20
Bleeding time, min	less than 7	2½	3	6
Prothrombin time, sec	12–15	13	13	13
Kaolin cephalin time, sec	35–55	55	80	150
Calcium thrombin time, sec	14–20	15	15	15
Factor VIIIC (iu/dl)	50–200	25	10	0
Factor VIIIRAg, %	50–200	122	150	230

Management

The mainstay of the treatment is the replacement of factor VIII.

Replacement therapy. Materials available are fresh frozen plasma, cryoprecipitate and freeze-dried human concentrate (Table 16.4). The half life of transfused factor VIIIC is between 8 and 12 hours and 60 to 90 per cent of the total dose given remains in the circulation after the infusion.

Fresh frozen plasma is prepared from freshly collected blood and stored at −30°C. A maximum of between 1–1·5 litres (15–20 ml/kg body weight) can be given; it produces a rise in factor VIII activity of 15–20 iu/dl. Fresh frozen plasma is only used when no other material is available: it may overload the circulation and cause serious allergic reactions.

Cryoprecipitate is prepared from individual freshly collected plasma donations. When plasma is frozen and then allowed to thaw below 8°C, fibrinogen, factor VIII and some other proteins remain forming an insoluble thick sludge or 'cryoprecipitate' at the bottom of the bag. The supernatant plasma is removed and the remaining 5–20 ml of cryoprecipitate refrozen at −30°C. Cryoprecipitate contains half to two thirds of the total factor VIII of the starting plasma and the usual final concentration is about 10–20 iu/ml. Before use, bags of cryoprecipitate are thawed at 37° and pooled together. As a dose for adults may require up to 30 or 40 bags, the preparation is time consuming and may involve significant loss of factor VIII. The dose of cryoprecipitate per kg of body weight varies according to the type of bleeding treated as shown in Table 16.4.

Freeze-dried concentrate of factor VIII (AHF concentrate). Concentrates of factor VIII are prepared by plasma fractionation. One type has about 5–10 iu per ml of final solution, and a second between 10–25 iu/ml. Some high purity preparations contain up to 300 iu/ml.

A rough assessment of amounts required and materials used can be made from data shown on Table 16.4. Ideally replacement therapy should be monitored with repeated factor VIIIC assays to ensure adequate factor VIII levels.

Table 16.4 Therapeutic levels of factor VIIIC related to the lesion treated, dose infused and material used

Lesion	Initial factor VIIIC level desired (iu/dl)	Dose of factor VIIIC iu/kg body weight)	Material
Minor spontaneous bleeding, haemarthroses, muscle haematoma	10–20	10–15	Cryoprecipitate Concentrate
Severe haemarthroses Minor surgery	30–40	20–30	Cryoprecipitate Concentrate
Major surgery	80–100	50–80	Concentrate

Spontaneous bleeding and minor haemarthrosis usually require one or two doses 24 hours apart. Such treatment soon relieves pain and the joint should be exercized immediately. *Major bleeding* into joints may require higher doses of factor VIII for up to five days. Immobilization is often required until pain and swelling have subsided. Physiotherapy is started as soon as possible. Very *large tense effusions* into joints may require aspiration, covered by factor VIII infusion; the factor VIII level should be raised to between 3 and 5 iu/dl.

In *dental extractions* the oral use of epsilon-aminocaproic acid (EACA) in a dose of 6 g or Cyclokapron 1 g every six hours, greatly reduces the amount of factor VIII required. The patient should be observed for a week. *Major surgery, orthopaedic procedures* or *extensive trauma* should be covered with high activity factor VIII concentrate to produce an initial factor VIII level of 80 iu/dl and keep it above 30 iu/dl during healing. Treatment is continued until healing, mobilization, removal of sutures and physiotherapy are complete. *Haematuria* and ureteric colic usually respond to treatment with factor VIII preparations if they raise factor VIII levels above 50 iu/dl.

Home treatment is satisfactory in selected cases. Parents or patients themselves inject the factor VIII kept at home. In this way early treatment is achieved; it provides more freedom for patients, although a close link with a haemophilia centre or hospital must be preserved.

Prophylaxis in severe haemophilia A is still controversial. Some good results are reported with factor VIII injections every 7–10 days. Such treatment maintains factor VIII at about 1–10 iu/dl and changes the clinical course of a severe haemophiliac into that of a moderately affected one with fewer bleeding episodes.

Complications of haemophilia and its treatment

Inhibitors of factor VIII. Six to seven per cent of haemophiliacs develop antibodies to factor VIII following treatment. These antibodies rapidly inactivate transfused factor VIII *in vivo* but the antibodies have proved difficult to demonstrate by immunological methods. They are IgG immunoglobulins and may either totally inactivate factor VIII activity or the complex of inhibitor with factor VIII may retain some clotting activity. An antibody unit has been defined as the amount of antibody (inhibitor) that will destroy 0·5 iu/ml of factor VIII after four hours incubation at 37° C.

The treatment of a haemophiliac with inhibitor is difficult. Antibody (inhibitor) production after transfusion of factor VIII will increase sharply within a week in most cases. Thereafter the antibody concentration slowly decreases over the next 3–9 months. Treatment requires large doses of factor VIII during the 4–7 days that precede the rise in antibody. With more than 5 u of antibody/ml it is rarely possible to achieve neutralization of antibody, although such patients still benefit clinically from treatment. Immunosuppression, plasmapheresis, concentrates of factor IX containing partially activated factors, and steroids have been used in reducing inhibitor levels.

Both *hepatitis* and the incidence of hepatitis-associated antigen and antibody is increased in patients with haemophilia. *Allergic reactions* have been described in patients receiving cryoprecipitate.

Other aspects of management. Patients with haemophilia should not be given aspirin or any antiplatelet drugs nor should they be given intramuscular injections. Good dental care is important. The patient or his parents should be given explicit instructions when to come to hospital for treatment. Appropriate explanatory booklets are available. Advice in relation to transport, holidays and career should be provided. All this is available in specialized Haemophilia Centres where prompt and appropriate replacement treatment is given.

Abnormalities of factor VIII—von Willebrand's syndrome

Von Willebrand's disease or syndrome is due to lack or to an abnormality of a plasma constituent, von Willebrand's factor, that is needed for normal cessation of bleeding and normal platelet function. These patients have a prolonged bleeding time and reduced levels of factor VIII activity. It is inherited as an autosomal dominant with varying expression and penetrance and affects both sexes equally.

Bleeding manifestations. Many patients with von Willebrand's syndrome are only *mildly affected*. They have nose bleeds, menorrhagia, bruising, occasionally gastrointestinal bleeding or epistaxis, as well as excessive blood loss after surgery or childbirth. In more *severely affected* patients with low factor VIIIC levels, bleeding into joints and muscles starts after the first year of life. Menorrhagia is particularly troublesome.

Diagnosis. The defect in von Willebrand's syndrome affects platelets as well as factor VIII. A combination of prolonged bleeding time and low plasma factor VIIIC levels are characteristic of von Willebrand's syndrome. Although the nature of the defect is as yet unclear, some of the recent observations such as low levels of Factor VIIIRAg and

Table 16.5 Coagulation tests in patients with von Willebrand's syndrome

Test	Normal	von Willebrand's syndrome	
		Mild	Severe
Whole blood clotting time, min	2–7	5	15
Bleeding time, min	7	9	>15
Prothrombin time, sec	12–15	14	14
Kaolin cephalin time, sec	35–55	49	78
Calcium thrombin time, sec	14–20	15	16
Factor VIIIC iu/dl	50–200	40	12
Factor VIIIRAg, %	50–200	46	0
Platelet retention by glass bead column, %	5–65	28	4
Platelet aggregation to ADP	N	N	N
collagen	N	N	N
ristocetin	N	Absent	Absent

impaired platelet agglutination to ristocetin, an antibiotic that causes agglutination of normal platelets, can be used to establish the diagnosis. (Table 16.5.)

Another useful diagnostic feature is that patients with von Willebrand's syndrome show a prolonged and progressive rise in factor VIIIC after infusion of small amounts of factor VIII or even of haemophilic plasma. Factor VIIIRAg does not show a similar rise and disappears promptly from the circulation. Recently *variants* of von Willebrand's syndrome with normal or even high factor VIIIRAg levels have been described. In these patients agglutination to ristocetin was impaired and the factor VIIIRAg had an abnormal electrophoretic mobility.

Management. Replacement therapy with fresh frozen plasma or cryoprecipitate is required for the more severely affected patients as in haemophilia. Sustained levels of factor VIIIC in plasma are usually easier to maintain than in haemophiliacs. The treatment should probably be started 2–3 days before operation to achieve maximum levels at the time of surgery and special attention should be paid to ensuring good local haemostasis. Severe menorrhagia can often be controlled with oral contraceptives. Rarely it is necessary to perform a hysterectomy or induce an artificial menopause.

Factor IX deficiency (Christmas disease)
Clinically factor IX deficiency or haemophilia B is indistinguishable from haemophilia A. Like haemophilia A it is a sex-linked recessive disorder, affecting males. The proportion of female carriers with mild bleeding manifestations is somewhat higher than in haemophilia A. One in five patients with haemophilia has haemophilia B.

Variants. Factor IX antigen is present in many patients in the absence of coagulation activity. In addition some patients suffering from haemophilia B show prolonged prothrombin times with ox brain thromboplastins such as Thrombotest, and they are said to have haemophilia B_m. Haemophilia B Leiden is a variant described in Holland where the manifestations of the disease become less severe at puberty with increasing levels of factor IX. Factor IX Chapel Hill has defective activation and is associated with mild disease.

Bleeding manifestations and the results of basic coagulation tests, except in haemophilia B_m, are identical to those in haemophilia A and the two can only be distinguished by carrying out correction tests with plasma from known cases or by performing specific assays.

Management. Replacement therapy with plasma or freeze dried concentrate is necessary for control of spontaneous haemorrhages and as cover for surgery. The factor IX concentrates contain factors X and prothrombin, and one type also has factor VII. Management is similar to that described in haemophilia A and virtually identical increases in factor IX concentration in plasma are required. Factor IX is much more stable than factor VIII *in vitro* and its plasma half life is longer, 18–30 hours; however, recovery of factor IX in the patient's blood after infusion is poor and shows marked variation from patient to patient (from 20–60 per cent of the original dose). Plasma (15–20 ml/kg of body weight) can be used to arrest spontaneous bleeding. The maximum rise of factor IX in a patient's circulation after plasma infusion is 5–10 per cent. When higher levels in plasma are needed as in surgery, dental extraction or more severe bleeding, factor IX concentrate is used. The levels of factor IX are kept at above 25 per cent until wounds have healed. This requires infusions of 30–60 units per kg of body weight every 24 hours. One unit is equivalent to the activity of one ml of average fresh normal plasma.

Home treatment and prophylactic treatment have been carried out with success. For prophylaxis in severely-affected individuals 2–3 injections of 20–40 u/kg are given twice weekly.

Factor VII deficiency

This is an uncommon, autosomal recessive disorder. The affected individuals have factor VII levels of less than 10 per cent. The only laboratory abnormality is a prolonged prothrombin time. The

Table 16.6 Laboratory findings in congenital clotting factor deficiencies other than haemophilia A and von Willebrand's syndrome.

Deficiency	One stage prothrombin time	Kaolin cephalin time	Thrombin time	Specific assay
Factor IX	Normal	Prolonged	Normal	Factor IX assay
Factor VII	Prolonged	Normal	Normal	Factor VII assay
Factor X	Prolonged	Prolonged	Normal	Stypven time, Factor X assay
Prothrombin	Prolonged	Prolonged	Normal	Prothrombin assay
Factor V	Prolonged	Prolonged	Normal	Factor V assay
Factor XI	Normal	Prolonged	Normal	Factor XI assay, Contact activation test
Factor XII	Normal	Prolonged	Normal	Factor XII assay, Contact activation test
Fibrinogen	Prolonged or normal	Prolonged or normal	Prolonged	Fibrinogen estimation, (thrombin clottable and immunological)
Factor XIII	Normal	Normal	Normal	Clot solubility in 5M-urea or acetic acid

bleeding manifestations are usually mild. The defect can be corrected by plasma infusion (10–15 ml/kg daily) or by using factor IX concentrate containing factor VII. The half life of factor VII is only 2–4 hours, but fortunately adequate haemostasis is achieved at levels of 5–10 per cent of the normal.

Factor X deficiency

This is a rare bleeding disorder inherited as an autosomal recessive. The defect varies from patient to patient suggesting that different molecular abnormalities of factor X occur. The bleeding manifestations are usually mild. Laboratory abnormalities (Table 16.6) include prolongation of the prothrombin time, partial thromboplastin time and stypven time in most cases. Bleeding can be treated by plasma (10–15 ml/kg daily) or factor IX concentrates. The half life of factor X is about two days and the haemostatic levels are about 10–20 per cent of the normal.

Prothrombin deficiency

Prothrombin deficiency is exceptionally rare. It can be due to either true hypoprothrombinaemia or to the presence of an abnormal prothrombin. Five families with an abnormal prothrombin have been described and these prothrombins are named prothrombin Cardeza, Barcelona, Padua, San Juan and Brussels. The bleeding manifestations are usually mild and are treated with factor IX concentrate, or plasma (15–20 ml/kg).

Factor V deficiency

Factor V deficiency is a rare mild bleeding disorder. In four cases an inhibitor of factor V appeared after plasma infusion. Replacement treatment can be given by infusing fresh plasma or fresh frozen plasma (15–25 ml/kg daily). Relatively low levels of factor V are required for haemostasis.

Factor XI deficiency

This is an uncommon incompletely recessive disorder affecting mostly those of Jewish origin. The bleeding manifestations are usually mild, and diagnosis may be difficult to establish. Factor XI deficiency is probably also a spectrum of different abnormalities, and plasma half life of factor XI was found to vary in different patients from 10–84 hours. Plasma (10–20 ml/kg body weight) or cryoprecipitate supernatant (10 ml/kg body weight) are usually required pre-operatively, with a maintenance dose of 5 ml/kg body weight daily every second day for a week or two.

Factor XII deficiency

Factor XII or Hageman factor deficiency is inherited as autosomal recessive trait. Most patients do not have a bleeding tendency, and some, including the original patient, Mr Hageman, have died from thromboembolic complications. Laboratory findings are identical to those for factor XI deficiency, and the diagnosis must be confirmed by carrying out correction tests with plasma from a proven case. In the few patients with a haemorrhagic tendency, surgery was covered by infusions of either stored, fresh or fresh frozen plasma.

Disorders of fibrinogen

These rare congenital disorders may be due to either an absent, a low concentration or an abnormal fibrinogen, afibrinogenaemia, hypo-fibrinogenaemia, and dysfibrinogenaemia, respectively.

Afibrinogenaemia is a rare autosomal recessive abnormality characterized by total absence of fibrinogen in plasma. The bleeding tendency is usually less than in a patient with severe haemophilia A. All the coagulation tests are abnormal. Liver function tests and individual factor assay are within the normal range but no fibrinogen is detectable in plasma. It is of interest that small amounts of fibrinogen can be demonstrated in the patient's platelets. When required fibrinogen is given. Levels above 0·6 g/l are haemostatic. The dose is 1·0 g per 10 kg body weight initially, and then 150 mg per 10 kg body weight daily in the treatment of bleeding or to cover surgery. Cryoprecipitate (2 ml/kg on the first two days of treatment and then 1 ml/kg) can also be used.

Congenital hypofibrinogenaemia. About 30 cases of this disorder have been described. A mild bleeding disorder exists in these individuals and the only abnormality is the reduced level of plasma fibrinogen.

Congenital dysfibrinogenaemia. These are autosomal dominant disorders characterized by the presence of functionally abnormal fibrinogens in plasma. The commonest defect is in the polymerization of fibrin monomers, although some abnormal fibrinogens show delayed cleavage of fibrin peptides. The affected individuals may be asymptomatic or show mild haemorrhagic or thrombotic tendency. In two families wound healing was found to be impaired. Laboratory diagnosis is not easy as the pattern is different from family to family. Usually a prolonged thrombin time and kaolin-cephalin time are present. All other tests may be normal. Fibrinogen levels estimated by clotting techniques give much lower results than fibrinogen levels estimated by physicochemical or immunological methods.

Deficiency of factor XIII

This is an inherited haemorrhagic disorder due either to lack of factor XIII or to the presence of non-functioning molecules of factor XIII in plasma and in platelets. The mode of inheritance is autosomal recessive. The patients have protracted bleeding from wounds starting 24–36 hours after injury. Bleeding from the umbilical stump during the first week of life is common. Joint bleeds, intracranial haemorrhage and recurrent spontaneous abortion are a feature in some patients. Poor wound healing may occur.

All screening tests are normal. However, the patient's clots are soluble in 5M urea and in monochloracetic acid. For detection of carriers more elaborate tests are needed, based on the incorporation of labelled amines.

Replacement therapy is easy because of the small quantities needed for haemostasis and the long plasma half life (3–6 days). The effect of a single (2–3 ml/kg body weight) injection of plasma lasts for up to one month. For this reason, prophylactic treatment with plasma or cryoprecipitate every 2–3 weeks has been successful. Abnormal wound healing has also been corrected by plasma infusions.

References

Austen D E G 1979 The structure and function of factors VIII and IX. Clinics in Haematology 8: 31–52

Biggs R 1979 Recent advances in the management of haemophilia and Christmas disease. Clinics in Haematology 8: 95–114

Nilsson I M 1974 In: Haemorrhagic and Thrombotic Diseases. John Wiley and Sons, London

Nilsson I M, Holmberg L 1979 Von Willebrand's disease today. Clinics in Haematology 8: 147–168

Rizza C R 1977 Clinical management of haemophilia. British Medical Bulletin 33: 225–230

Rizza C R, Biggs R 1973 The treatment of patients who have factor VIII antibodies. British Journal of Haematology 24: 65–81

17

Acquired disorders of coagulation

Many diseases are associated with abnormalities of haemostasis. The bleeding manifestations of liver and kidney disease, myeloproliferative disorders and myeloma are described in appropriate chapters. This chapter deals with disseminated intravascular coagulation, circulating anticoagulants, and the haemorrhagic manifestations of cardio-pulmonary by-pass and the post-perfusion period.

Disseminated intravascular coagulation (Defibrination syndrome)

Disseminated intravascular coagulation (DIC) is due to widespread activation of coagulation in the blood. This results in consumption of coagulation factors and platelets, fibrin deposition and secondary fibrinolysis. DIC is always secondary to other diseases (Table 17.1). It may occur as an acute, fulminant bleeding disorder or as a more chronic condition with both haemorrhagic and thrombotic manifestations.

In acute DIC there may be a sudden onset of purpura, bleeding

Table 17.1 Conditions sometimes associated with DIC.

Acute

Shock	Burns
Septicaemia	Major surgery, especially thoracic
Acute intravascular haemolysis	Bites of some poisonous snakes
Abruptio placentae, amniotic fluid embolism, septic abortion	Heat stroke
Acute pulmonary embolism	Cardiac arrest and resuscitation
Acute liver failure	

Chronic

Disseminated malignancy	Aortic aneurysm
Pancreatic carcinoma	Giant haemangioma or haemangioblastoma
Promyelocyte leukaemia	
Retained dead fetus	

from the gastrointestinal, urinary or genital tract, from operative wounds, oozing from venepunctures and injection sites and formation of large tracking bruises. Blood loss, hypovolaemic shock and fibrin deposition in the renal micro-circulation may lead to acute renal failure due to renal cortical necrosis. A combination of haemorrhagic and ischaemic changes in the skin sometimes results in purpura fulminans or even gangrene. Some patients show evidence of DIC in laboratory tests but do not bleed. This may occur in septicaemia and concealed accidental haemorrhage. In patients with chronic DIC, especially in malignancy, thrombotic manifestations such as recurrent deep venous thrombosis or embolization from large non-bacterial vegetations on heart valves may predominate.

Pathogenesis
DIC can be triggered directly by clot-promoting substances entering the circulation (trauma, amniotic fluid embolism, snake venom), or indirectly by toxic agents (endotoxins, antigen-antibody complexes) damaging red cells, leucocytes, platelets or vessel walls to release clot-promoting substances. Factors that predispose to DIC are abnormalities of the mononuclear-phagocytic system, liver disease, pregnancy and reduced fibrinolytic activity.

The haemostatic abnormalities occurring in DIC are shown schematically in Figures 17.1 and 17.2. The release of clot-promoting

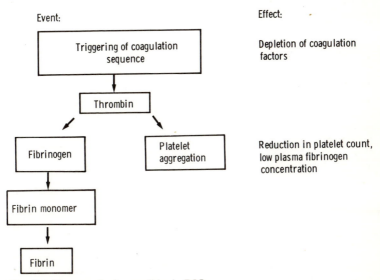

Fig. 17.1 Haemostatic abnormalities in DIC.

substances into the circulation results in the *generation of thrombin.* Thrombin splits fibrinopeptides A and B from fibrinogen, and fibrin monomers are formed. This leads both to the reduction in the levels of plasma *fibrinogen,* and to *fibrin deposition* with formation of circulating *fibrin monomer complexes* with fibrinogen (Fig. 17.1). The deposition of fibrin in the micro-circulation provokes brisk *secondary fibrinolysis* (Fig. 17.2). This in turn may lead to an increased concentration of *fibrin-fibrinogen degradation products* (FDP). FDP may complex with fibrin monomers and cause further impairment of clotting. The combined effects of thrombin and plasmin on factors VIII, V and prothrombin, and to a lesser extent on XI and XII, cause *depletion* of these factors in the circulation. *Platelets* are aggregated and deposited in the micro-circulation where widespread thrombin generation and fibrin deposition occurs; they are also involved as a part of the triggering mechanism. The bleeding in DIC is the result of lack of coagulation factors, thrombocytopenia and anticoagulant effect of FDP.

Red cells become entrapped in the fibrin mesh laid down in the micro-circulation and may get fragmented while passing through it. In some cases the damage to red cells is so severe that a haemolytic anaemia occurs.

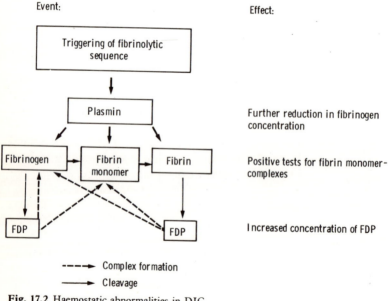

Fig. 17.2 Haemostatic abnormalities in DIC.

Diagnosis

The initial tests carried out in a bleeding patient are the prothrombin time, kaolin-cephalin time, calcium thrombin time and platelet count. The first three tests are prolonged and the platelet count reduced. Thereafter fibrinogen and FDP concentration are measured and the presence of fibrin monomer complexes looked for. The diagnosis of chronic DIC can be difficult as results of tests may be normal or only slightly abnormal. The condition is suspected in the presence of a persistently high FDP concentration, positive fibrin monomer test and a reduced platelet count. The typical findings in an acute and a chronic case are shown in Table 17.2.

Table 17.2 Laboratory findings in patients with DIC

		DIC	
Test	Normal	Acute	Chronic
Prothrombin time. sec	12–15	45	17
Kaolin cephalin time. sec	35–55	90	28
Calcium thrombin time. sec	14–20	>60	22
Platelet count/ × 10⁹/l.	150–400	20	80
Fibrinogen g/l	1·5–4·0	0·4	8·2
Fibrin monomer complex	Negative	Positive	Positive
FDP μg/ml	2·5	1200	80

Management

Treatment of the causative disease such as removal of a dead fetus, treatment of septicaemia or hypovolaemic shock removes the triggering mechanism. DIC itself may not require active intervention but treatment may be required to stop bleeding and to prevent tissue damage. Whole blood is used to replace the blood lost and prevent shock. Coagulation factors may be replaced with fresh frozen plasma. If cryoprecipitate or fibrinogen are given, the deposition of fibrin from the infused material may lead to further tissue damage. Nor should platelet concentrates be given in the acute phase as they may form aggregates that block the microcirculation. The fibrinogen level and the platelet count are monitored carefully during treatment.

Decision whether to give heparin, which can arrest intravascular coagulation, is difficult since there is the risk of provoking further bleeding. It has been used with success in amniotic fluid embolism, in acute promyelocytic leukaemia, malignancy with thrombotic manifestations, haemangioma, purpura fulminans and in haemolytic uraemic syndrome. If heparin is given low doses (maximum 10–15 iu/kg body weight/per hour) should be used, at least initially.

Fibrinolysis

Primary fibrinogenolysis is an extremely rare condition associated with liver disease or carcinoma of the prostate. There is systemic fibrinolysis without activation of coagulation. It should be suspected in a patient with laboratory signs of DIC but with normal platelet count and extremely short euglobulin or dilute whole blood clot lysis time.

Local fibrinolysis is thought to be one of the causes of bleeding after prostatectomy or bladder operations. Endometrium has a very high plasminogen activator content and increased fibrinolytic activity is one of the contributory causes of menorrhagia. Local fibrinolysis plays an important role in further bleeding after subarachnoid haemorrhage.

Synthetic antifibrinolytic agents (epsilon-aminocaproic acid and tranexamic acid) have been used to suppress local fibrinolysis in these conditions. Both drugs are rapidly absorbed from the gastrointestinal tract and excreted in urine. The concentration of EACA in urine is 80–100 times that of plasma. Usual doses are 20–30 g EACA or 2–6 g tranexamic acid per day by mouth. The main danger is formation of unlysable clots in the urinary tract and thrombosis.

Circulating anticoagulants

Circulating anticoagulants are acquired inhibitors of blood coagulation present in blood which directly inhibit clotting factors and their reactions. The commonest anticoagulant is directed *against factor VIII* and is a complication of severe haemophilia (Ch. 16). Some individuals with normal factor VIII levels develop an inhibitor to factor VIII. It can appear after parturition, or in patients suffering from immune disorders such as rheumatoid arthritis, asthma, severe penicillin allergy as well as in those with no underlying disease.

The clinical manifestations are the same as those in severe haemophilia. The laboratory findings are also identical to those in haemophilia, and the presence of the circulating anticoagulant can be demonstrated by the inhibitory effect of the patient's plasma on normal plasma. Occasionally the circulating anticoagulant may disappear spontaneously, but more usually the prognosis is poor, especially in the elderly.

Management of bleeding is by replacement with high purity factor VIII concentrate, or with factor IX concentrates containing activated coagulation factors. Although there is often no rise in factor VIII plasma concentration, the bleeding may stop. Corticosteroids and immunosuppresant drugs, in particular cyclophosphamide, as well as plasmapheresis, have been used in the treatment of this condition.

Some patients with *disseminated lupus erythematosus* develop a circulating anticoagulant that interferes with prothrombin conversion to thrombin. Most of these patients do not bleed excessively and the abnormality is detected by a prolonged prothrombin time and kaolin-cephalin time. Mixing tests show that the patient's plasma prolongs the prothrombin time and the kaolin-cephalin time of normal plasma. Patients with disseminated lupus erythematosus who bleed usually have thrombocytopenia and low prothrombin levels in addition to the anticoagulant. The anticoagulant may persist indefinitely in untreated patients, but disappears on steroid therapy.

An inhibitor of fibrin stabilization causing a severe haemorrhagic diathesis has been described after transfusion and in rare patients taking isoniazid.

Haemorrhagic manifestations of cardiopulmonary by-pass

Haemorrhage is a frequent and serious complication in the use of an extra-corporeal circulation. During the perfusion bleeding is usually due to the presence of heparin and to the reduced platelet count. The post-perfusion bleeding is usually to result of inadequate neutralization of heparin, but is sometimes caused by thrombocytopenia or disseminated intravascular coagulation, usually in patients after a long perfusion with low cardiac output. The effects of massive blood transfusion may also produce adverse effects. Investigation must establish whether or not heparin has been neutralized and if not, the calculated dose of protamine is given. The platelet count is invariably low ($20-60 \times 10^9/l.$). Fresh frozen plasma and platelet concentrates should be used to correct the depletion of clotting factors and platelets.

Table 17.3 Laboratory tests in acute acquired bleeding disorders.

Condition	Platelet count	Prothrombin time	Kaolin-cephalin time	Calcium thrombin time
DIC	low ($20-50 \times 10^9/l.$)	prolonged	prolonged	very prolonged
Massive transfusion	low ($40-80 \times 10^9/l.$)	prolonged	prolonged	normal
Liver disease	low	very prolonged	prolonged	prolonged
Heparin	normal	prolonged	prolonged	prolonged
Circulating anticoagulant	normal	normal	prolonged	normal
Undiagnosed congenital deficiency	normal	normal	prolonged	normal

Investigations in a patient with an acute acquired bleeding disorder
There is usually little time for complicated tests. Information for diagnosis and treatment is obtained from the platelet count, prothrombin time, kaolin-cephalin time and calcium thrombin time. Blood should be collected into EACA-citrate to enable reliable determination of fibrinogen and fibrin-degradation products at a later stage. Results are shown in Table 17.3.

References

Bowie E J W, Owen C A Jr 1977 Hemostatic failure in clinical medicine. Seminars in Haematology 14: 341–364

Nilsson I M 1974 Haemorrhagic and thrombotic diseases. John Wiley and Sons, London

Shapiro S S 1979 Antibodies to blood coagulation factors. Clinics in Haematology 8: 207–214

18

Malignant blood diseases

Preleukaemic syndrome
Leukaemia
The Leukaemic cell
Chronic lymphocytic leukaemia
Acute lymphoblastic leukaemia

Prolymphocytic leukaemia
Leukaemic reticulo-endotheliosis
Myeloma
Chronic myelocytic leukaemia
Acute myeloblastic leukaemia

The preleukaemic syndrome
In a small proportion (less than 10 per cent) of patients in whom myelomonocytic leukaemia appears, the disorder is preceded by a rather ill-defined blood disorder which antedates the manifestations of leukaemia by between three months to three years. There are non-specific symptoms of weakness and lassitude and in some, weight loss and bruising. Slight enlargement of liver and spleen occurs in about 15 per cent.

The blood count shows a moderate anaemia, often macrocytosis, neutropenia, thrombocytopenia and a 'monocytosis'. Agranular neutrophils may be present. The marrow is usually of increased cellularity, there may be megaloblastosis not reversed by folate or cobalamin, sometimes ringed sideroblasts but generally there are no firm diagnostic features. Follow up of this refractory anaemia shows the emergence of leukaemic features, usually within two years.

Leukaemia—general comments
Leukaemia is a neoplastic disease of haemopoietic cells. The chronic forms have a clinical duration of several years and involve a proliferation of mature or maturing blood cells. The acute forms have a clinical duration of months, if left untreated, and involve proliferation of immature blood cells. In both there is progressive infiltration and replacement of normal bone marrow by leukaemic cells and a general infiltration of tissues throughout the body.

Diagnosis is made by the demonstration of the leukaemic cells, either immature or mature, in blood and/or marrow. There are many classifications of leukaemia, particularly as a greater understanding of their relationships emerge, and the one that follows is based on the appearance of these cells in the stained blood and marrow film.

The clinical features and the management of the disease are discussed under the different disorders. Some of the features of the leukaemic cell are described in the next section.

Table 18.1   The leukaemias

Chronic	—	Myelocytic (granulocytic)
		Lymphocytic
Acute Myeloid	—	Myeloblastic
		Myelomonocytic (Naegeli)
		Promyelocytic
		Erythroleukaemia (Di Guglielmo)
		Smouldering
Monocytic	—	(Schilling)
Lymphocytic	—	Acute
		Prolymphocytic
Undifferentiated	—	

The leukaemic cell

Morphology. Inspection of a peripheral blood and marrow film is the first step in morphological diagnosis of leukaemia. One attempts to relate the leukaemic cell to its counterpart in normal blood and marrow and on this basis the disorders may be grouped as indicated in Table 18.1.

Granules in the cytoplasm and Auer rods (azurophil rods probably lysosomal in nature) indicate a myeloid origin. They do not occur in lymphoblastic leukaemias. The company the cell keeps is always of great importance. The presence of granules in some cells indicating a tendency to develop to promyelocytes suggest that the blast cells are myeloblasts. A myelocyte failing to make granules looks like a monocyte but in these cases granules may be present in marrow cells. Maturation of a myelocyte in the absence of granule formation leads to agranular neutrophils, an important sign in early leukaemia.

Prolymphocytic leukaemia differs in morphology, clinical features and prognosis from chronic lymphocytic leukaemia. The cell has one or more distinctive nucleoli and is accompanied by a very high total white cell count.

There are many acute leukaemias that cannot be pigeon-holed into these rough categories on the basis of their morphological features.

Electron microscopy has added little but has helped in the characterization of cell organelles (granules, rods etc.) and is useful in confirming a rare variant of the lymphocyte called leukaemic reticuloendotheliosis or hairy-cell leukaemia, the latter descriptive title referring to fimbria arising from the cell membrane.

Cytochemistry. The results that may be expected with cyto-chemical staining techniques are shown in Table 18.2.

Sudan black and peroxidase stains should be positive in acute myeloblastic leukaemias. The periodic acid Schiff reaction should give a coarse or block positive reaction in the cytoplasm in about 70 per cent of cases of acute lymphoblastic leukaemia.

An acid phosphatase reaction is positive in leukaemic reticuloendotheliosis (hairy-cell leukaemia) but results vary with different substrates.

The leucocyte alkaline phosphatase shows a strong positivity in myeloproliferative disorders but leukaemic cells react weakly or are negative. Some of the methods are difficult to apply and results are often not very helpful.

Table 18.2   Cytochemistry in acute leukaemia.

	Lymphoblastic	Myeloblastic	Myelomonocytic	Ethyraemic myelosis
PAS	coarse +	fine ±	±	±
Sudan Black	−	± to + +	+	+
Peroxidase	−	± to + +	−	+
Esterase*	− or ±	±	+	+
Auer rods	−	+	+	+

*results vary with substrate employed

Chromosomes. The philadelphia chromosome is the name applied to the abnormal chromosome present in 92 per cent of patients with chronic myelocytic leukaemia. It is chromosome G22 which has lost a portion of its long arm which has been translocated, usually to C9, but in 8 per cent of cases to other chromosomes. Sometimes chronic myelocytic leukaemia presents for the first time in the terminal phase which is a blast cell crisis. This phase can be distinguished from other acute leukaemias by the presence of the philadelphia chromosome.

About half the patients with acute leukaemias have normal chromosomes and no consistent abnormality has been demonstrated in the remainder. In acute myeloblastic leukaemia the abnormalities disappear with remission of the disease unlike chronic myelocytic leukaemia where the philadelphia chromosome persists.

Surface markers. The great majority of lymphocytes in chronic lymphocytic leukaemia are B-lymphocytes although often the cells only show weakly positive reactions with some reagents, for example for complement receptors, while being negative with others. IgM and IgD are the commonest immunoglobulins on the cell surface and they are all of the same light chain type indicating their monoclonal origin. Other results are shown in Table 18.3. The majority of cases of childhood lymphoblastic leukaemia are neither of B-nor T-type but have been termed null-cells. But 20–30 per cent are T-cells and these constitute a poor prognostic group and very few (2–3 per cent) are B-cell leukaemias.

An antiserum has been prepared against the common acute lymphoblastic leukaemia antigen and this reacts with almost all the null-cell types as well as with cells from some cases of blast cell crisis in chronic myeloid leukaemia. Another antigen detected in these cells has been termed Ia.

Enzymology. Lysozyme (muraminidase) levels in blood and urine are higher in acute leukaemias with monocytic features. Adenosine deaminase activity is elevated in acute lymphoblastic leukaemias.

Terminal deoxynucleotidyl transferase (TdT) is normally present only in cells of the thymus gland and is a hallmark of the early lymphoblast, possibly a stem-cell. The enzyme is present in about 95 per cent of cells from acute lymphoblastic leukaemia and in cells from about one third of patients with a blast cell crisis in chronic myeloid leukaemia. Such cases are sensitive to treatment with vincristine-prednisone.

The presence of steroid receptors on the cell surface has also proved to correlate well with clinical responsiveness to steroid therapy.

Table 18.3 Cell surface markers in leukaemia

Type of leukaemia	B–cell %	T–cell %	Null–cell %
Chronic lymphocytic	+95	2–3	–
Prolymphocytic	90	10	–
Reticuloendotheliosis	100	–	–
Acute lymphoblastic	2	20–30	70–80
Sezary syndrome	100	–	–
Lymphosarcoma with spill over	70	30	–
Burkitts' lymphoma	100	–	–

Chronic lymphocytic leukaemia

All patients with this disorder have in common an absolute increase in the number of lymphocytes in blood. Lymphocytes in chronic lymphocytic leukaemia are essentially the same in appearance as those seen in normal blood, that is, they may be of the small lymphocyte or large lymphocyte variety. The latter cell with nucleoli is sometimes called a 'prolymphocyte'. An additional feature seen in blood films from patients with chronic lymphocyte leukaemia is that many lymphocytes are disrupted in the process of spreading the film and these are called smear cells. This disruption is prevented by spreading the blood film in a drop of AB serum or bovine albumen.

Lymphocyte numbers are higher in children than in adults, the range being 4000–10 000/μl in the first year of life, 2000–8000/μl up to the age of four, and up to 5000 till the age of about seven. Thereafter the absolute lymphocyte number should not normally exceed 4000/μl.

An increase in lymphocyte numbers is a feature of many disorders in children and with the exception of glandular fever, only rarely a feature of disease in adults. Lymphocytosis occurs in:

1. Pertussis (whooping cough), acute infectious lymphocytosis, glandular fever (EB virus, cytomegalic virus, toxoplasmosis).
2. Chronic lymphatic leukaemia.
3. Acute lymphoblastic leukaemia.

A percentage increase in lymphocytes in many other diseases reflects a neutropenia without any significant change in lymphocyte numbers and emphasizes the importance of thinking in terms of absolute numbers of cells in the differential count. This applies to many virus diseases such as hepatitis, measles, rubella and mumps.

Clinical. Chronic lymphocytic leukaemia occurs in the last few decades of life, 90 per cent of patients being over the age of 50. It is more common in men than women. The wide variety of presentation illustrates many of the clinical problems.

1. Unexpected lymphocytosis in a blood count performed for other reasons is one of the ways in which symptom-free cases are detected. There is virtually no other cause of a persistent absolute increase in lymphocytes in an adult other than chronic lymphatic leukaemia. The total lymphocyte level is often between 5000–30000/μl but may be much higher.
2. The patient may go to see his doctor because of the appearance of lumps—enlarged lymph glands on the neck, axillae and groin. He may feel perfectly well and have no other complaints.
3. The patient may present with the signs and symptoms of severe anaemia sometimes accompanied by bruising. The marrow in such patients is heavily infiltrated with lymphocytes. Apart from the absolute lymphocytosis the blood shows a pancytopenia. The lymphocyte increase may be modest not exceeding 10000/μl or may be very high even in excess of 100000/μl. The blood lymphocyte level does not necessarily bear any relationship to the severity of the disease or to its manifestations.
4. The patient may present to the dermatologist with a generalized raised erythematous skin disorder due to lymphocytic infiltration of the skin.
5. The patient may have an autoimmune haemolytic anaemia with a positive direct antiglobulin test (Ch. 13).

6. The patient may present with repeated serious infections, often of the chest, due to grossly impaired immunological capacity.
7. There may be enlargement of salivary glands and lymph glands—so called Mikulicz syndrome.
8. The patient may present with Raynaud's phenomenon with cold pale cyanosed extremities (hands, feet, ears, nose) due to a cryoglobulin—an abnormal protein precipitating out of solution in the cold.

Examination may not show any abnormal findings in early cases. In others there may be enlarged lymph glands in one or several sites and this may be accompanied by splenomegaly. Eventually enlarged glands appear and gradually increase in size and spleen and liver continue to enlarge. Mediastinal, mesenteric and retroperitoneal glands may be involved.

Histologically there is widespread tissue infiltration with lymphocytes and this is responsible for the varied manifestations of this disease. Mitoses are infrequent since the disease involves an increasing accumulation of long-lived lymphocytes.

A useful staging procedure has been proposed by Rai *et al* as follows.

Stage 0   Lymphocytosis only, in excess of $15\,000/\mu l$.
Stage I   Lymphocytosis with lymphadenopathy.
Stage II   Lymphocytosis with enlarged spleen or liver. Glands may or may not be enlarged.
Stage III Lymphocytosis with anaemia. Liver, spleen or glands may or may not be enlarged.
Stage IV   Lymphocytosis with thrombocytopenia. Liver, spleen or glands may or may not be enlarged.

Median survival of patients in Stage 0 is greater than 150 months, Stage I 101 months, Stage II 71 months, Stage III 19 months and Stage IV 19 months.

Patients found to have an elevated lymphocyte count alone may show little change for many years. Others with some of the other manifestations have a more aggressive form of the disease which may require repeated intervention or may follow a fairly rapid downhill course. The natural history is so variable that prognosis should be guarded.

Aetiology. Virtually nothing is known about causative factors. A few families in whom several cases of chronic lymphatic leukaemia developed have been described. Rarely chromosomal abnormalities have been recorded. The vast bulk of cases do not show such features. There is no relation to radiation.

Haematology. Peripheral blood shows an absolute lymphocytosis with a varied proportion of smear cells. This may be accompanied by anaemia, thrombocytopenia and/or neutropenia. Spherocytes with polychromasia will characterize those cases in whom there is an autoimmune haemolytic anaemia.

The marrow even in the mildest cases contains increased numbers of lymphocytes—generally the number of lymphocytes in a normal marrow depends on whether the needle is in the region of a lymphoid follicle or not, but in a normal marrow it is unusual for more than 20 per cent of cells to be lymphocytes. Less commonly the marrow is packed with lymphocytes and a dry tap may result. Serial trephine indicates that this develops from the coalescence of enlarging lymphoid follicles in the marrow. A packed marrow indicates a relatively poor prognosis. Such cases may have severe anaemia with reduction in platelets and neutrophils. They do not tolerate cytotoxic drugs very well and resotration of normal haemopoiesis, which depends on eliminating lymphoid cells from the marrow, may prove difficult.

Immune status. Chronic lymphocytic leukaemia has been described aptly as an accumulation of immunologically-incompetent lymphocytes. This may manifest itself clinically by a marked susceptibility to recurrent infections which often prove fatal. This includes susceptibility to bacterial infections such as pulmonary infections, tuberculous infection which may be disseminated (miliary) and viral infections including herpes zoster, hepatitis, encephalitis, etc. Infections, particularly viral, tend to be disseminated rather than local.

The vast majority of lymphocytes in chronic lymphocytic leukaemia that can be characterized, behave as B-cells. The numbers of T-cells probably remain unchanged though considerably diluted by the large excess of B-cells. In addition there are a large number of cells which do not have immunoglobulins on their surfaces, nor do they form rosettes with sheep cells. They are probably defective B-cells since some have complement receptors on their surface.

Low serum levels of immunoglobulins (hypogammaglobulinaemia) are present in 35–50 per cent of all patients. This may affect all the immunoglobulin classes, but sometimes only IgA is reduced. Humoral antibody responses, particularly to injections of pneumococcal polysaccharide, are reduced and antibodies present in most normal sera such as those against *E. coli* or staphylococci, are often absent.

Cell-mediated immunity is equally impaired and this can be demonstrated by a negative tuberculin skin test and failure to react to mumps or candida antigens given intradermally. Stimulation with DNCB (2,4-dinitrochlorobenzene) fails to produce a response. Many of the lymphocytes are inert, failing to undergo mitosis normally when incubated with phytohaemagglutinin.

In addition to depressed immunological function abnormal immunoglobulins may be present. These are detected generally by their clinical effects as well as in the laboratory. Some 5 per cent of patients have a monoclonal immunoglobulin in either the β or γ region on serum electrophoresis and this is either IgA, IgG or IgM. As in myeloma the M protein is generally associated with depression of normal immunoglobulins.

Less commonly proteins precipitating in the cold (cryoglobulins) are present. An autoimmune haemolytic anaemia may be the presenting feature in about 5 per cent of patients (Ch. 13) and such patients may have only a modest increase in blood lymphocytes as the only evidence of chronic lymphocytic leukaemia, although others may have more advanced disease.

Diagnosis depends on demonstrating an absolute persistent lympho-cytosis in blood. The appearance of the lymph gland in lympho-sarcoma (non-Hodgkin's lymphoma) and lymphatic leukaemia is the same but in lymphosarcoma immune capacity is usually retained whereas in chronic lymphatic leukaemia it is usually defective.

Management. There is no curative treatment. Management is designed to keep the patient comfortable. Treatment is required when the disease threatens health; occasionally to remove unsightly glands.

In practice this means that many patients do not need treatment at all. Such patients usually have an elevated lymphocyte count, possibly some moderately enlarged glands and a normal haemoglobin level. Such patients should be followed checking both the blood and their clinical state six-monthly.

Occasionally unsightly glands in the neck may be treated with local X-ray therapy. Patients with repeated infection and hypogamma-globulinaemia may benefit from gammaglobulin replacement therapy given as regular injections. There is a tendency to start treatment at an earlier stage of the disease and some will start treatment in patients at stage I of the Rai classifications and almost all will treat stage II.

Steroids such as prednisone (40 mg/day) are indicated in patients with autoimmune haemolytic anaemia and in those with anaemia and a packed marrow and should be continued for at least 4–6 weeks and then replaced by a cytotoxic agent.

Chlorambucil is the most widely used drug. The starting dose varies from 4–10 mg daily (0·2 mg/kg/day). It may be continued for six or more weeks at this level and is followed by a smaller maintenance dose. Chlorambucil may be added to steroids if the effects of steroids are too slow or inadequate and it should overlap steroid therapy in those requiring longer term maintenance. Cyclophosphamide may be used instead of chlorambucil. Intermittent 5 day courses with steroids repeated at 4–6 weekly intervals are often equally effective (Chlorambucil 10–20 mg daily and prednisone 40 mg daily).

Response occurs over several weeks with reduction in lymphadenopathy and fall in blood lymphocyte numbers. Splenomegally however, may persist for a long time. Marrow infiltration is often resistant to therapy although there is a significant improvement in blood values which may even become normal. Such patients are treated more vigorously with the type of regime used in lymphoma, for example, courses of cyclophosphamide, vincristine and prednisone with or without adriamycin, (CHOP or COP).

Adverse effects of prolonged use of steroids are stimulation of protein breakdown (thinning of skin with striae, muscle wasting, osteoporosis with fractures), cushinoid changes (rounding of face, hirsutes), diminshed carbohydrate tolerance, acne, adrenal suppression and immunosuppression. Occasionally gastric haemorrhage, precipitation of diabetes, oedema, psychoses and amenorrhoea may follow prolonged use.

The main adverse effect of chlorambucil is marrow depression with neutropenia and thrombocytopenia. Cyclophosphamide in addition to toxic effects on the marrow, may cause alopecia (loss of hair) and haemorrhagic cystitis.

Acute lymphoblastic leukaemia

This is the common acute leukaemia of childhood. Its incidence is highest in the first five years of life. An apparent increase in frequency of this disorder over the last 30 years is probably due to the control of intercurrent infections with antibiotics which in the past led to the death of such children before underlying leukaemia was apparent.

Unusually acute lymphoblastic leukaemia occurs in adults. The frequency in children is 1 in 3000. About 90 per cent of childhood leukaemias are lymphoblastic and 10 per cent myeloblastic. The distinction between these two forms of leukaemia is important because patients with the myeloblastic form have a poor outlook.

Aetiology
Genetic factors play a significant but uncertain role. Thus if one of a pair of identical twins has leukaemia there is a one in five chance that

the second identical twin will also show evidence of leukaemia within the next few months. There is an association between certain disorders characterized by *chromosomal abnormalities* and leukaemia. This applies to mentally-defective children with mongolism (Down's syndrome) where the chance of leukaemia is one in 95, as well as to patients with Fanconi's anaemia and Bloom's syndrome. In Down's syndrome there is an abnormal chromosome 21. In the other disorders there are chromosomal breakages.

Radiation exposure is a predisposing factor to leukaemia. This was established by the studies of survivors of atomic bomb explosions in Japan where an increased frequency of acute lymphoblastic as well as acute and chronic myeloid leukaemia, occurred. Diagnostic X-ray procedures in the mother at the stage of the early embryo doubles the chance of leukaemia in the offspring.

Viral factors. Leukaemia in the chick, mouse and rat is caused by a virus which can be isolated from the animal. These virus particles will induce leukaemia in other susceptible animals. Burkitt's lymphoma is a malignant disease of lymphoid tissue occurring in children in certain parts of Africa and New Guinea but in virtually no other parts of the world. Even in these tropical areas it only occurs above a certain altitude. The disease itself bears many similarities to acute lymphoblastic leukaemia. The geographical distribution of Burkitt's lymphoma could be accounted for if an insect-borne virus were involved. There is an association between Burkitt's lymphoma and the Epstein-Barr virus. In addition a type C virus particle was obtained from a cell line originating from a Burkitt's lymphoma. Such C-type particles have been associated with RNA tumour viruses.

In other parts of the world the occurrence of unexpected 'clusters' of cases of leukaemia in small localities has been thought to be suggestive of infectious agent. More recently a bone marrow transplant from a male donor was carried out successfully in a girl with acute lymphoblastic leukaemia. The girls own cells had first been destroyed by irradiation. When the leukaemia recurred the 'new' leukaemic cells were of the XY or male donor type. This suggests that an agent such as a virus had maintained the leukaemic process in the new, hitherto unaffected, normal donor cells.

Further data which suggest how a viral agent might act has come from studies on reverse transcriptase. Mammalian virus-induced tumours contain a viral RNA sequence and an enzyme, reverse transcriptase, which together result in the synthesis of tumour DNA. Such RNA and reverse transcriptase have been identified in blood cells from 95 per cent of all types of human leukaemia but not from normal human blood cells. These abnormal RNA sequences persist in the blood from patients with lymphoblastic leukaemia long after the patient is in full remission. This work suggests that successful treatment returns the growth pattern of leukaemic cells to normal rather than eradicates the leukaemia.

Clinical aspects

The disease appears insidiously and the parents will indicate that the child has not been well for 4–6 weeks, sometimes longer. The commonest symptoms are those of anaemia, that is, listlessness, and weakness. The parents may note the accompanying pallor. Half the children may have bled unduly either into skin or from the nose. Sometimes infection is present—chest, ear or mouth. Bone pain is not uncommon. Less commonly, enlarged lymph glands are noted. Headaches and vomiting may occur.

On examination there may be pallor, ecchymoses and purpura. Enlarged lymph glands and enlarged spleen (up to 5 cm below the costal margin) usually with an enlarged liver are present in $\frac{3}{4}$ of the children. Sternal tenderness may be present.

Blood and marrow. The blood count generally shows a low haemoglobulin concentration and a low platelet count. In the majority of patients the total white cell count is either normal or reduced. In about one-third the total white cell count is increased and occasionally it is very high. The predominant cell is a lymphoid cell with a fairly finely patterned chromatin, a very thin rim of cytoplasm and either no nucleoli or some ill-defined nucleoli. Occasionally round vacuoles are present in the cell. It does not have the very fine chromatin texture and sharply defined nucleoli of the myeloblast and in fact, looks like a fleshy lymphocyte.

Marrow may be difficult to aspirate but fluid from the marrow needle shows sheets of uniform 'blast' cells. These cells are early haemopoietic cells related to the lymphoid series. They usually show block positivity in the PAS stain and 70–80 per cent are null cells, most of the remainder being T-cells. Most show terminal transferase (TdT) activity (see earlier section).

Management

The objective of treatment in lymphoblastic leukaemia in childhood is to produce a clinical cure. As a result of many clinical trials on the efficacy of various regimens a relatively standard therapeutic approach has evolved that produces a remission in about 85–90 per cent of children and an apparent cure in more than 50 per cent.

1. Treatment is started with Vincristine (1·5 mg/sq metre body surface intravenously once weekly for 4–6 weeks) and Prednisone (40 mg/sq metre body surface daily by mouth for 4–6 weeks). These two drugs do not depress marrow function, unlike almost all other drugs used in treatment of cancer, and act quickly so that steady improvement in platelet and neutrophil levels are evident within days. This limits the need for additional supportive measures. The addition of a third drug, either L-asparaginase or daunarubicin increases the remission rate from over 80 per cent to between 90–95 per cent of children so treated, and reduces the number who relapse subsequently. After the fourth week, if the peripheral blood is normal a marrow is carried out. If the marrow still shows evidence of leukaemia, treatment is carried out for two more weeks. At the end of this period if the marrow is now normal in appearance the next stage is started (Table 18.4).

Table 18.4   Regime for treatment of acute lymphoblastic leukaemia

Remission induction
Prednisone	–	40 mg/sq metre/day orally for 28 days
Vincristine	–	1·5 mg/sq metre/week i.v. for 4 weeks
Daunarubicin	–	25 mg/sq metre/week i.v. for 4 weeks

Central nervous system prophylaxis when remission is achieved
Cranial radiation for 2½ weeks
2400 rads for children over 2 years of age
2000 rads for children 1–2 years of age
 500 rads for children less than 1 year of age
Intrathecal methotrexate – 12 mg/sq metre twice weekly
 for 2½ weeks coincident with cranial irradiation.

Maintenance therapy for 30 months
6–mercaptopurine	–	5 mg/sq metre/day orally
Methotrexate	–	20 mg/sq metre/week orally

2. In order to 'eliminate' residual leukaemic cells from the nervous system (brain and spinal cord) the skull is irradiated. This may result in temporary loss of hair. At the same time a lumbar puncture is carried out twice weekly and Methotrexate is given intrathecally each time until five doses have been given.
3. Thereafter, the patient is placed on a drug regime for three years consisting of 6-mercaptopurine daily and Methotrexate weekly.

Blood counts and marrow examinations are carried out regularly throughout this period. If there is no relapse, treatment is stopped after 2½ to 3 years.

More than half the children who do not relapse during the three-year treatment do not show further evidence of disease after cessation of treatment. Often the maintenance treatment is interrupted by marrow depression and/or a sore mouth. The toxic drug is the Methotrexate and the dose will be reduced or even omitted for one or more weeks to allow marrow recovery. These children are severely immunosuppressed and a few succumb from rapid overwhelming infection although in full haematological remission. This description applies to the uncomplicated case. Some children may be very anaemic on presentation or have severe bleeding manifestations or be infected and appropriate supportive therapy may be required (see myeloblastic leukaemia).

Children who fail to respond to Vincristine-Prednisone should have other cytotoxics added. The most important additional drug is probably Cytosine arabinoside. A regime termed COAP (cyclophosphamide, Oncovin = vincristine, Ara—C = cytosine arabinoside and prednisone is often used. When remission is obtained the regime discussed above is pursued. Other drugs and regimes are discussed in relation to acute myeloblastic leukaemia.

Central nervous system involvement. Before cranial irradiation was instituted about one half of the children with acute lymphoblastic leukaemia developed CNS relapse while the blood was still in remission. This was due to failure of anti-leukaemic drugs to penetrate the meninges and CSF. The appreciation that this site was the source of leukaemic cells responsible for relapse, led to the use of 'prophylactic' irradiation. Meningeal leukaemia is associated with a raised intracranial CSF pressure and the appearance of blast cells in the CSF. The commonest complaints are headache, vomiting and lethargy. There may be papilloedema (fluid exudate in the retina obscuring the normally sharp outline of the optic nerve), accompanied by disturbances of vision (double vision, squint, blurring), nerve paralyses and irritability. Treatment is to instil 5 mg Methotrexate into the CSF on alternate days until abnormal cells disappear. Relief of the CSF pressure usually produces prompt relief of symptoms and other manifestations generally disappear rapidly. However, several episodes of meningeal leukaemia may occur in the same patient during the course of the disease.

Family discussion. A discussion with both parents about the implications of the disease, the prognosis and management is necessary. If the child enquires about the diagnosis it should be given in a straightforward factual manner. The child should continue normal activity as far as possible without any special concessions being made. Favoured treatment invariably antagonizes other siblings and produces tensions in the family.

Other aspects of management are discussed in relation to myeloblastic leukaemia. Haematological relapses should be treated with vincristine—prednisone and if necessary other drugs. There is a high likelihood of second and third remissions.

Prognosis is best in children with relatively low total white cell counts and without clinical enlargement of organs. These probably have a lower leukaemic cell mass than those with high white cell counts and heavy organ infiltration. Children, often boys older than 5 years, with a white cell count greater than 20 000/μl and whose cells show the characteristics of T-lymphocytes are likely to relapse and should be treated more energetically than outlined in this discussion. The median WBC count at diagnosis in this group is 100 000/μl and three-quarters have mediastinal lymphadenopathy.

Adults with lymphoblastic leukaemia do not do as well as children and are better treated in a manner similar to acute myeloblastic leukaemia.

Prognosis is also better in girls because there is a recurrence of leukaemia in the testes in between 8–16 per cent of boys in various series and this occurs some three years after initial diagnosis (range 3–66 months). It is treated with local irradiation.

Prolymphocytic leukaemia

This is a rare disease of older people. In addition to lassitude there may be a tendency to bruise easily. On examination there is considerable splenomegaly without any enlargement of lymph glands.

There is anaemia and a very high total white cell count often exceeding 200 000 per μl. The vast majority are prolymphocytes with one to three very sharply delineated nucleoli.

Prognosis is poor but some have benefitted in the short term from splenic irradiation and others from cytotoxic drugs (CHOP regime). Most die from thrombotic complications.

Leukaemic reticuloendotheliosis (hairy-cell leukaemia)

This is another rare disorder of the elderly. The patient often presents with general ill-health and the blood count shows a pancytopenia which unless the haematologist shows unusual perspicuity, defies diagnosis. If the spleen is not palpable on presentation, it becomes so over the months. Small numbers of atypical lymphoid cells may be present in peripheral blood and marrow.

The diagnosis is made by suspecting that such cases may be hair-cell leukaemia and taking steps to detect the fimbriated appearance of the cell surface, and seeking confirmation with an acid phosphatase reaction which should be tartrate resistant.

A variety of treatments have been tried including splenectomy followed by steroids and/or cytotoxic drugs. Some show marked benefit.

Myeloma

This disorder is due to a diffuse, rarely to a localized, marrow infiltration with plasma-type neoplastic cells. These abnormal cells secrete an abnormal plasma protein. Its frequency increases with age, being uncommon below the age of 50.

Other than an increase in myeloma following irradiation due to atomic explosions in Japan its cause is not known.

Clinical aspects. The majority of patients have bone pain as the dominant symptom. Most commonly this is a low back pain. Collapse of vertebrae may lead to pressure on nerves causing both pain and neurological manifestations including paraplegia. Some patients show an increased susceptibility to infection; others a bleeding diathesis due to complexing of abnormal protein with coagulation factors or to coating of platelets; and others evidence of impairment of circulation such as blindness, the result of a very high plasma viscosity. Occasionally the discovery of an abnormal protein in plasma or the investigation of protein in urine, may reveal an asymptomatic case.

Examination. This may reveal areas of bone pain. Other findings may relate to bone collapse. There may be evidence of renal failure with drowsiness.

Radiology. X-ray may show clear translucent punched-out areas where myeloma has eroded bone. There may be collapse of vertebral bodies, sometimes with a marked thinning out of the spine (osteoporosis). These osteolytic lesions tend to progress.

Blood and marrow. The haemoglobin concentration may be reduced but often this is due to a markedly increased plasma volume with haemodilution. This in turn is due to an increased osmolarity, the result of the high plasma protein concentration, which draws in and holds additional fluid in the plasma compartment.

The blood film characteristically shows intense rouleaux with background staining due to the raised plasma protein level. Occasionally normoblasts, myelocytes and plasma cells are seen. The ESR is very high. The sternum may be fragile in myeloma and very little pressure may be needed to penetrate cortical bone in performing a marrow aspiration.

The marrow may show sheets of myeloma cells with relatively few cells of other types. In other cases there may be abnormal numbers of cells of myeloma type and in some just increased numbers of cells indistinguishable from normal plasma cells. Less commonly, the marrow may be normal. The myeloma cells differ from plasma cells in that they have distinct nucleoli and they may be pleomorphic, that is, they may have marked variation in cell appearance and multi-nuclearity. Rheumatoid arthritis and related disorders may be associated with increased plasma cell numbers. Thus sometimes the marrow can only be described as compatible with myeloma.

Abnormal proteins. A characteristic feature of myeloma is the presence of abnormal proteins in blood and/or urine. In serum electrophoresis this appears as a distinct spike in the β–γ region—so-called monoclonal globulin (M-protein). In half the patients this M-protein is an IgG immunoglobulin and in about 20 per cent it is an IgA. Uncommonly IgM is present and about 25 per cent do not have an M-protein, but have only Bence-Jones protein. Bence-Jones protein is the light chain portion of the immunoglobulin molecule. Classically this protein in urine is precipitated with heat when the temperature reaches about 50–60°C and re-dissolves at about 90°C. Light chains are looked for by immunoelectrophoresis against kappa and lambda antisera after concentrating the urine. Light chains are present in urine in about 75 per cent of patients with myeloma.

The serum albumin concentration may be abnormally reduced. The levels of normal immunoglobulins IgG and IgA may be low rendering the patient very liable to infection which is often a terminal event. Renal function is often damaged due to deposits of protein in renal tubules so that the blood urea is high. Bone destruction releases large amounts of calcium so that plasma calcium is abnormally high. This by itself produces further renal damage so that death from uraemia is common.

Diagnosis. This depends on demonstrating the myeloma and/or their products which are M-proteins and/or light chains. Radiological evidence is helpful but can be due to other neoplasms.

Management. The purpose of management is to relieve pain and to prolong life by slowing the growth of myeloma where possible. Not all patients with a paraprotein require treatment. In many, particularly in elderly patients, the course of the disease for a long time follows a relatively benign course. These patients cannot be identified with certainty but those who have just an M-protein with or without evidence of abnormal cells in the marrow, should be watched. Pain, light chains in urine, bony lesions on X-ray, raised serum calcium and anaemia are indications for therapy.

Elevation of plasma calcium levels requires urgent treatment with rehydration of the patient by encouraging intake of fluids, and prednisone (40 mg/day) to reduce serum calcium by encouraging its excretion into the urine. Investigations which lead to dehydration are avoided and in particular, an intravenous pyelogram is dangerous since it may precipitate irreversible renal failure. Local pain or collapse may be treated with local irradiation. An orthopaedic back support may also be helpful.

Two drugs have proved to be of value in about half the patients. Melphalan (10 mg daily by mouth for seven days, repeated every 6–8 weeks). This is often combined with prednisone (40 mg/day for seven days). The second drug is Cyclophosphamide which is given at a dose level of 200 mg daily by mouth for seven days followed by 50–100 mg daily for maintenance, and which is as effective as Melphalan. When successful there is disappearance of pain over the course of a few weeks, followed by decline in the level of M-protein and great improvement in mobility.

Melphalan (phenylalanine mustard). This is usually well tolerated but sometimes may produce some nausea and vomiting. Overdosage can produce marrow depression. Long term use invariably results in macrocytosis with a raised MCV.

Prognosis depends on renal function and on whether the myeloma is responsive to therapy. An elevated blood urea and low serum albumin indicate a poor outlook.

Chronic myelocytic leukaemia

This is a disorder characterized by a marked increase in granulocytes in blood and marrow, splenomegaly and a characteristic chromosomal translocation.

Aetiology. It arises as a result of a mutation affecting the haemopoietic stem cell so that a new clone bearing the imprint of the chromosomal abnormality replaces normal cells in the blood and marrow. Further evidence for the clonal origin of this disease comes from observation of negro females (sex chromosome XX) heterozygous for a variant of the X-linked enzyme, glucose-6-phosphate dehydrogenase, who also developed chronic myeloid leukaemia. These women had a type B G6PD enzyme (on one X chromosome), and an A variant common in negroes, transmitted on the other X chromosome. In each cell one of the X-chromosomes is normally suppressed, i.e. in each cell either the A enzyme or B enzyme is present. In a mixture of cells, for example from a skin biopsy, both types are detected. In the patients with chronic myeloid leukaemia fibroblasts grown from their skin showed both A and B enzymes whereas chronic myeloid leukaemia cells showed only one enzyme suggesting an origin of the leukaemia from a single cell.

As with the acute leukaemias radiation exposure is an aetiological factor, that is, there was an increased incidence after nuclear bomb explosions, in radiologists and in those exposed to therapeutic irradiation of the spine for ankylosing spondylitis.

The other major abnormality in chronic myeloid leukaemia is the loss of much of the longer arm of chromosome 22 and its translocation usually to chromosome 9. The abnormal chromosome 22 is referred to as the Philadelphia or Ph' chromosome. All typical examples of chronic myeloid leukaemia have the Ph' chromsome, and it is present in all haemopoietic cells in this disease but not in other tissues.

Clinical aspects. This is a disease of adult life with a peak incidence between 20–60 years of age. The earliest evidence of the disease is an increasing elevation of the WBC count with immature forms in the stained films, followed by enlargement of the spleen.

Patients complain of tiredness, sweating and loss of weight. The fully developed case is anaemic with a white cell count of the order of $200\,000/\mu l$ and a very large spleen comparable in size to that seen in chronic myelofibrosis. Bone tenderness is quite common.

Diagnosis. This is straightforward. The total white cell count is very high and the differential count includes myeloblasts, promyelocytes and myelocytes of all types and at all stages of development, as well as mature cells. An increase in basophils is common and only occurs in myeloproliferative disorders. The platelet count is often raised and may exceed one million/μl. Occasionally it is abnormally low. Anaemia is the rule in the untreated well established case and normoblasts may appear in the blood.

Marrow is of greatly increased cellularity with marked granulo-poietic activity and many megakaryocytes.

Other findings are an elevated blood uric level and a very high serum vitamin B_{12} level of several thousand pg/ml due to a very high level of transcobalamin I binder in plasma. The Philadelphia chromosome is present in granulocytes, megakaryocytes and erythroid cells in both marrow and peripheral blood preparations in all typical cases. Leucocyte alkaline phosphatase level tends to be low.

Management. The purpose is to reduce the white cell count to near normal levels and maintain it at these levels. As this is achieved there is a reticulocytosis with return of the red cell count to normal and clinical improvement including disappearance of the enlarged spleen. Irradiation of the spleen produces prolonged remissions although overall survival is probably better with cytotoxic drugs. The most widely used drug is busulphan (2–6 mg daily) both for inducing remission and maintenance, but Melphalan, Cyclophosphamide, Chlorambucil, 6-mercaptopurine, Thioguanine, Hydroxyurea and Dibromomannitol are all effective though less easy to use than busulphan. The blood count must be followed closely and the drug stopped in anticipation of the white count reaching normal levels. Overtreatment with busulphan may lead to fatal aplasia.

Even in good remission the blood cells remain Ph' chromosome positive. Survival after diagnosis averages about 3–4 years.

Blast-cell crisis. The vast majority of patients who do not die of some intercurrent event, enter the final phase of the disease. It may be suspected by the white cell count continuing to rise despite increase in the dose of drug, by lack of clinical well being, by an increase in the proportion of blast cells in the differential white cell count and by a falling haemoglobin concentration.

In about a third of blast-cell transformations the cells have lymphoid characteristics both in appearance, in their possession of a terminal transferase (TdT) enzyme and in their responsiveness to vincristine and prednisone even though this response is very short lived. In the rest the morphology is that of a myeloblastic leukaemia. At this stage survival is not likely to be more than several weeks as worthwhile remissions are unusual.

It has been suggested that when the patient first presents marrow be stored in liquid ntrogen and when the terminal blast-cell crisis develops, the acute leukaemia population be eliminated with cytotoxic drugs, and white cells from the chronic phase be returned to the patient to re-establish the chronic phase. This has been done with success in several patients.

Philadelphia chromosome negative cases. These patients (about 10 per cent of the total) are more difficult to treat and have a much shorter survival.

Childhood granulocytic leukaemia. These are generally Ph' chromosome negative. In young children (age 1–2) this is a more acute disease with intercurrent infection, bleeding, difficulty in control with cytotoxics and a fatal outcome usually within months. They have a raised HbF level.

In older children a more typical Ph' chromsome positive disease may occur which behaves like the adult form.

Acute myeloblastic leukaemia and its variants
This is a neoplastic proliferation of early granulocytic cells. Causative

factors have been discussed under acute lymphoblastic leukaemia. A variety of chromosomal abnormalities occur in about half the patients but these are the result of leukaemia and disappear in remission. Following atomic explosions in Japan, cases of acute leukaemia first appeared within two years and the peak incidence was reached 5–7 years later.

A factor which permits survival of abnormal leukaemic cell clones is loss of normal immune responses. It is presumed that potentiallly neoplastic cell clones are produced from time to time and are normally eliminated. In immunosuppressed patients, e.g. those being treated with long term cytotoxic drugs, such clones may persist. Thus a significant incidence of tumours including leukaemia develops in such patients.

Variants of granulocytic leukaemia are largely based on morphological differences but these different types do show some clinical differences as well. Those types are:

acute granulocytic leukaemia;
acute promyelocytic leukaemia;
acute myelomonocytic leukaemia;
acute monocytic leukaemia;
erythroleukaemia;
myelomonocytic or smouldering leukaemia of old age.

Clinical aspects. There are over 35 deaths due to acute leukaemia per 100 000 population each year and the highest frequency is in the oldest age groups. The patient goes to the doctor because of shortness of breath and lethargy due to anaemia, because of bruising and bleeding due to lack of platelets (or coagulation factors), or because of infection due to lack of neutrophils and failure of the normal immunological responses to infection. Far less commonly, he or she will notice enlarged lymph glands, a skin rash due to infiltration with leukaemic cells or be referred by a dentist because of swollen spongy bleeding gums.

Examination may show pallor, bruising and purpura, mouth ulceration and swollen gums (a feature of monocytic and myelomonocytic leukaemia). There may be a raised temperature. Lymph glands and spleen may be enlarged. Infection and haemorrhage are the main causes of death.

Blood. Anaemia, a low platelet and neutrophil count are the rule. The total white cell count is variable being low, normal or high. Failure of development of granules in neutrophils is a common feature and suggestive of leukaemia in 'early' cases. In myeloblastic leukaemia the myeloblast is usually the predominant cell, having a fine chromatin pattern, several well developed nucleoli, and, on adequate search, Auer rods.

In monocytic and myelomonocytic leukaemia, the predominant cell may be a so-called, monocyte—almost invariably this is an agranular myelocyte—that is, a myelocyte in which granules have failed to develop. In acute promyelocytic leukaemia the majority of leukaemic cells are promyelocytes. Erythroleukaemia shows a mixture of myeloblasts and abnormal erythroblasts with megaloblastic features and irregular and often multiple nuclei.

In old people a more benign version of myelomonocytic leukaemia is common, characterized by some anaemia, variable but usually low platelet count, agranular neutrophils often in adequate numbers, and agranular myelocytes.

Marrow. The marrow in acute leukaemia is usually of markedly increased cellularity being packed with early granulocytic precursors. Often when the peripheral blood has many monocytes the marrow shows similar cells with some granulation indicating their granulocytic rather than their monocytic origin. In the myelomonocytic leukaemia of old people the marrow is often of normal cellularity with an increase in the proportion of myeloblasts. In promyelocytic leukaemia again the marrow is filled with promyelocytes and similarly in erythro-leukaemia, both myeloblasts and bizarre erythroblasts predominate.

It is generally believed that true monocytic leukaemia exists. Other terms used in the literature such as plasma cell leukaemia, eosinophilic and basophilic leukaemia are variants of myeloma and chronic myelocytic leukaemia, respectively.

Special stains are discussed earlier in this chapter.

In a leukaemoid reaction there is a large increase in numbers of neutrophils and late myelocytes in the blood. This occurs in infections or neoplasms and their differentiation from leukaemia is not a real problem. It must be remembered that patients with leukaemia have low resistance to tuberculosis which may become active and even disseminate. A 'leukaemic' blood picture in tuberculosis is almost certainly an associated true leukaemia and not a leukaemoid reaction. Occasionally acute leukaemia presents as a refractory anaemia. Marrow shows an increased proportion of blast cells but is of normal cellularity.

Coagulation findings. Evidence of disseminated intravascular coagulation is common. In promyelocytic leukaemia there appears to be release of thromboplastic material by the promyelocytes which initiates variable changes in coagulation factors. In addition to raised fibrin monomers there may be low fibrinogen, factor V and VIII levels.

Management

Some current regimes of treatment are probably more unpleasant for the patient than the disease itself and judgement as to whether to proceed to induce a remission should be tempered with mercy. In many older patients it is better to give palliative treatment and aim at keeping the patient comfortable. The myelomonocytic leukaemia of old people (sometimes called 'smouldering' leukaemia), progresses only slowly over several years.

The objective of therapy is to induce a haematological and clinical remission. To this end a combination of cytotoxic drugs are given to produce transient marrow aplasia. This phase of marrow aplasia is accompanied by pancytopenia and supportive therapy is needed. About 40–50 per cent of adults then show a return of normal blood formation, but with experience many groups are now obtaining a 70 to 80 per cent remission rate with a cytosine/thioguanine/daunarubicin regime. The remainder die during this phase or show a return of leukaemic cells to the marrow. Remission may last up to a year, occasionally longer and in this phase blood and marrow may appear normal. Relapse is heralded by an increase in leukaemic cells in the marrow followed by their reappearance in the blood. A second and even third remission can be induced in some patients.

Supportive treatment. Red cells are transfused as required and fresh platelet concentrates are given to prevent bleeding. A few centres have the facility to concentrate and transfuse white blood cells and these may prove valuable in combating otherwise resistant infection.

Prevention of infection is the most important problem in management. This concerns not only common bacterial pathogens but rare pathogens such as Pneumocystis carinii. Fungal infections (candida) may become widespread. Gram-negative organisms such as pseudomonas may produce septicaemia with collapse of the patient. Some centres attempt to set up a sterile environment for the patient, even supplying sterile food etc. Other centres sterilize the gastro-intestinal tract with antibiotics, such as Colistin and clean the skin with local bactericidal washes. Others accept that infection will need to be treated at some phase and nurse the patient in a general ward. In general these precautions reduce the incidence of infection but do not improve the remission rate. Severe infection may be accompanied by disseminated intravascular coagulation which may need replacement of coagulation factors in addition to platelets.

Antileukaemic therapy. Simultaneous use of a number of drugs has proved more effective than the use of single drugs. Some of these drugs are:

Cytosine arabinoside is a pyrimidine antagonist which interferes with the incorporation of cytosine into both DNA and RNA. It is given by injection and produces gross megaloblastic changes. In combination with one or more other drugs it is the mainstay of all successful remission-induction schedules.

Methotrexate is a folic-acid antagonist blocking the enzyme dihydrofolate reductase which converts dihydrofolic acid to tetra-hydrofolic acid. Dihydrofolic acid is normally generated in thymidine synthesis. Like cytosine arabinoside it is active against dividing cells and its toxic effects are marrow depression (via gross megaloblastic changes), mouth and gut ulceration and in the long term, cirrhosis of the liver. It is given by mouth.

6-mercaptopurine and *thioguanine* are purine antagonists, less toxic than the two previous drugs but can produce marrow depression. They are given by mouth.

Cyclophosphamide is an alkylating agent given orally or by injection. injection.

Vincristine is an alkaloid derived from the blue periwinkle. It is given by injection and interferes with the events of mitosis. It is most useful in lymphoblastic leukaemia. It can produce very severe constipation and peripheral neuritis which is reversed on drug withdrawal.

Daunorubicin (Daunamycin) is derived from growth of a strepto-myces strain. It is given by injection and is a powerful marrow depressant as well as damaging cardiac muscle.

Adriamycin (doxorubicin) is similar to daunamycin.

L-asparaginase breaks down asparagine required by tumour cells whereas normal cells are able to synthesize this aminoacid. It is

Table 18.5   Drug combinations used in treatment of acute leukaemia

Drug	COAP	TRAP	POMP	CART	OAP	DOAP	TAD
Prednisone	+	+	+		+	+	
Vincristine	+		+		+	+	
6–Mercaptopurine			+				
Thioguanine		+		+			+
Methotrexate			+				
Cyclophosphamide	+						
Cytosine-arabinoside	+	+		+	+	+	+
Daunarubicin		+		+		+	+
Asparaginase				+			

relatively toxic but useful in lymphoblastic leukaemia. *Prednisone* is toxic to lymphoid cells.

Of the drugs available cytosine arabinoside given alone produces remissions in 24 to 42 per cent of patients with acute myelocytic leukaemia and daunarubicin alone remissions in 43 to 50 per cent of treated patients. Given in combination the remission rate is significantly higher. A regime consisting of cystosine (100 mg/sq metre i.v.), thioguanine (100 mg/sq metre orally every 12 hours) for 7 days with daunarubicin (60 mg/sq metre i.v. on days 5, 6 and 7) has yielded an 80 per cent remission rate. Other regimes are shown in Table 18.5.

The median duration of remission is 7 to 10 months. Intensive therapy following the induction of remission (hopefully called consolidation) and varying regimes of maintenance therapy have produced only modest prolongation of remission or no prolongation at all.

Toxic effects of cytotoxic drugs

Marrow. Vincristine, L-asparaginase, bleomycin and steroids are marrow sparing. With busulphan the neutrophils continue to decline at least two weeks after the last dose. Most cytotoxics lead to macrocytosis.

Gastrointestinal tract. Nausea and vomiting for several hours and even days after administration of multiple cytotoxic drugs is very common. It may be ameliorated by prior administration of fluphenazine 1·5 mg and nortriptylline 30 mg daily. Mouth ulceration and painful throat is common with methotrexate and daunarubicin. It may be relieved by local anaesthetic lozenges such as lignocaine. Candidiasis is another complication, prophylactic nystatin or miconazole being used. Long term use of methotrexate is associated with a high incidence of cirrhosis. Cholestatic jaundice is an unusual complication of long term mercaptopurine.

Skin. Almost total loss of scalp hair occurs with cyclophosphamide, daunarubicin and doxorubicin although the hair regrows after cessation of therapy. A wig must be provided. Cytotoxics are normally injected through a rapidly running saline infusion and extravasation can cause considerable pain and ulceration at the drip site. Skin pigmentation has been reported with daunarubicin.

Nervous system. A peripheral neuropathy is common with vincristine affecting both motor and sensory paths. It can affect cranial nerves. Severe constipation requires prophylactic use of dioctyl and similar compounds. An atonic bladder and impotence may reflect autonomic neuropathy. These all reverse on cessation of vincristine therapy. Intrathecal methotrexate can produce meningeal irritation of short duration and rarely more severe brain damage.

Cardiovascular. Irreversible cardiotoxicity is a serious complication of daunarubicin and doxorubicin. Cardiac failure develops months after therapy and is related to the total dose given the upper limit being 750 mg/sq metre with daunorubicin and 600 mg/sq metre with doxorubicin.

Lungs. Pulmonary fibrosis manifested by increasing dyspnoea even at rest, is a rare complication of busulphan and even more rarely of cyclophosphamide.

Genito-urinary tract. High dose methotrexate can produce irreversible renal change. Rapid destruction of leukaemic cells can lead to high uric acid levels preventable by allopurinol. High doses of cyclophosphamide can produce a sterile haemorrhagic cystitis. Daunarubicin may cause red discoloration of urine following its excretion.

Other. Glycosuria and sometimes frank diabetes can be precipitated by steroids. This is usually reversed on withdrawal. Other effects have been mentioned.

Immunotherapy. More recently attempts have been made to stimulate an immune response by the host against the leukaemic cell. There are tumour-specific antigens on neoplastic cells which differ from antigens in normal cells but the patient with active malignant disease lacks normal immune responses. Non-specific stimulation with regular injections of BCG vaccine has been given as well as with blast cells collected and stored during the acute phase of the illness. It is uncertain whether these methods produce significant benefit.

Bone marrow transplantation. Patients with acute leukaemia who have an identical twin, have been treated with supralethal irradiation, cyclophosphamide, marrow transplant from their twin followed by immunotherapy with both normal twin lymphocytes and stored irradiated leukaemic cells. In at least nine cases the treated twin remained free of disease. Marrow transplants from non-identical donors have yielded 15 per cent long-term survivors at the time of writing.

References

Gale R P, Cline M J 1977 High remission-induction rate in acute myeloid leukaemia. Lancet 1: 497–499

Rai K R, Sawitsky A, Cronkite E P, Chanana A D, Levy R N, Pasternak B S 1975

Clinical staging of chronic lymphocytic leukaemia. Blood 46: 219–234
Roath S 1972 Acute leukaemia. Clinics in haematology. Saunders, London
Soarni M I, Linman J W 1973 Preleukaemia. Amer J Med 55: 38–48
Simone J V 1978 Acute leukaemia. Clinics in haematology. Saunders, London

19

The effect of systemic disease on the blood

Anaemia of chronic disorders

Anaemia is usual in many chronic diseases whether inflammatory, neoplastic or metabolic in nature. The anaemia is usually moderate in degree but on occasion may be more severe. These disorders include rheumatoid arthritis, renal and hepatic failure, tuberculosis, malignant disease and many others.

Apart from reduction in red cell count the blood may be unremarkable or it may resemble in some detail the blood in iron-deficiency anaemia. Thus the red cells are often microcytic with a low MCV, MCH and MCHC and the serum iron level is low. The anaemia differs from that in iron deficiency in that the serum iron-binding capacity is also low (it is high in iron deficiency) and that the marrow stained by Perls's method shows the presence of iron in macrophages.

A number of factors contribute to the development of the anaemia.

1. Failure of iron re-utilization. In this condition iron from broken down red cells tends to be retained in macrophages rather than released to the marrow for haemoglobin synthesis. As a result the serum iron level is low.
2. In many patients there is a modest shortening of the red cell life span due to factors outside the red cells since these cells survive normally in a healthy recipient. The mean red cell life span is rarely reduced below 30 days.
3. Inadequate marrow response. There is no increase in erythropoiesis in response to anaemia and this in turn, may be related to relatively low levels of erythropoietin although the marrow itself is capable of responding to the hormone.

Treatment is that of the underlying disease of which the anaemia is a manifestation.

Malignant disease

The changes in the blood in malignant disease may be those described under 'anaemia of chronic disorders', that is, there may be a moderate degree of anaemia and the red cells are either normal in size and appearance or they may be microcytic and hypochromic.

When the marrow is infiltrated with malignant cells, immature cells of both red and white cells series may appear in the blood. Anaemia with both myelocytes and normoblasts present in the stained blood film is called a leucoerythroblastic anaemia. The explanation for the release of immature cells is not clear. It may involve some marrow disorganisation or be due to the appearance of foci of blood formation outside the marrow such as spleen and liver (extramedullary haemopoiesis). The early cells may arise from these sites.

Malignant cells in marrow may be seen on marrow aspiration or trephine and may prove of clinical value in diagnosis.

Exceptionally malignant disease may be the cause of more unusual blood pictures. Thus if it is associated with disseminated intravascular coagulation fragmented red cells may appear. Neoplasia may be the cause of a haemolytic anaemia, of a leukaemoid blood picture and with the rare erythropoietin-producing tumours of a polycythaemia. Marked infiltration of marrow may lead to pancytopenia that must be distinguished from an aplastic anaemia.

Lead poisoning

This arises from an abnormally high intake of lead. It may occur in young children at the age when they tend to eat paint from walls or cot sides (pica), in those exposed to lead at work, or drinking or eating food cooked in pots with high lead content.

In adults anaemia is moderate in degree but may be more severe in children. The blood tends to be microcytic and hypochromic, there is polychromasia with an increased reticulocyte count and an increased number of the polychromatic cells show basophilic stippling.

The marrow may show both micronormoblasts (as in iron-deficiency) and ringed sideroblasts.

Lead interferes with haem synthesis and with the incorporation of iron into haem. Because there is a failure of utilization of protoporyphyrin, this compound accumulates in the red cells and coproporphyrin is excreted in excessive amount in faeces. There is also impaired conversion of delta—aminolaevulinic acid (ALA) into porphobilinogen and ALA is excreted into the urine.

The diagnosis may be suspected clinically (a history of exposure, colicky abdominal pain and a black line at the junction of gums and teeth—lead line), there may be a hypochromic blood picture with basophilic stippling and diagnosis is confirmed by measuring blood lead which is normally less than 40 μg/100 ml and is increased in lead poisoning.

Treatment is by removal of the source of lead contamination and if necessary, by agents which mobilize and excrete lead from the body (EDTA or penicillamine).

Major haemorrhage

Persistent loss of small volumes of blood leads to an iron-deficiency anaemia. Acute loss of a large volume of blood produces acute symptoms due to the sudden reduction in total blood volume.

Loss of 500 ml of blood as in a blood donation for transfusion purposes, produces few symptoms other than slight tiredness several hours later. When blood loss is 1000–1500 ml (20 to 30 per cent of blood volume) there is an increased pulse rate particularly on exercise, and even some fall in blood pressure on standing up. When blood loss approaches 2000 ml in an adult severe symptoms are present including faintness, a cold clammy skin, rapid shallow breathing and a rapid pulse rate. There is a fall in blood pressure. Larger bleeds are generally fatal.

A blood count taken shortly after a major bleed does not reflect the severity of blood loss which must be assessed on clinical grounds. It may take up to three days for plasma volume to be restored and to reveal the degree of anaemia (Fig. 19.1). A blood count taken a few days after a major bleed will show anaemia but red cells are normal in

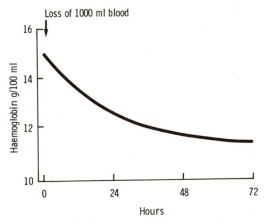

Fig. 19.1 Change in haemoglobin concentration after a 1000 ml haemorrhage.

appearance. There may be some polychromasia and even some normoblasts in the film, often with a neutrophil leucocytosis.

Clinical management is aimed at restoration of blood volume by transfusion of plasma-volume expanders in the first instance (dextran, plasma) and whole blood as soon as it is available.

Cardiac failure

Congestive cardiac failure is usually associated with poor oxygenation of blood. There is evidence of compensation by an increased haemoglobin concentration. Often in severe congestive cardiac failure there is polychromasia with raised reticulocyte count and normoblasts in the circulating blood. These latter findings disappear with treatment.

Congenital heart disease may be associated with shunting of blood away from the lungs and this produces a secondary polycythaemia. Such patients are usually cyanosed. Artificial heart valves may lead to a haemolytic anaemia due to mechanical damage to red cells (Ch. 13). Myocardial infarction is usually followed by a neutrophil leucocytosis first appearing within 4–5 hours and persisting for 3–4 days.

Disseminated lupus erythematosus (DLE)

This is an autoimmune disorder with very variable clincial manifestations such as joint pains, skin rash, malaise, fever, loss of weight, high blood pressure etc. The haematologist is often involved both through the effects on the blood as well as in demonstrating some of the phenomena such as L–E cells and anti-nuclear factor.

L–E cells are demonstrated by incubating a whole blood sample for several hours and then preparing stained films from the 'buffy' or white-cell rich layers. Sera from such patients contain an IgG immunoglobulin which reacts with free nuclear material converting this to homogeneous pink-staining balls. These are ingested by neutrophils giving the appearance of a polymorph nucleus and cytoplasm stretched around the rim of this ball (Fig. 19.2). Their presence is diagnostic of DLE including those forms occurring in response to drugs such as Procainamide, Hydrallazine and Practolol. It may occur in lupoid hepatitis and sometimes in rheumatoid arthritis. L–E cells must be differentiated from 'tart' cells which arise when a neutrophil engulfs a lymphocyte. In a tart cell the morphology of the lymphocyte nucleus remains relatively unaltered.

Antinuclear factor is detected by adding the patients serum to a frozen section of tissue such as liver. The antinuclear globulin will attach to the cell nuclei and this may be demonstrated by the addition of a fluorescein-labelled antiglobulin serum. Inspection with an appropriate microscope will show fluorescence over the nuclei. This test is more sensitive but less specific than finding of L–E cells. The agglutination by sera of latex particles coated with gammaglobulin is another test for anti-nuclear factor.

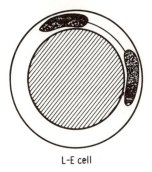

L–E cell

Fig. 19.2 An L–E cell.

Apart from these diagnostic measures the majority of patients with DLE are anaemic, a few severely (see page 223). About 1 in 20 patients with DLE come to clinical notice because of an autoimmune haemolytic anaemia and almost one third of all patients may have a positive direct antiglobulin test.

Thrombocytopenia is another manifestation of DLE and is managed in essentially the same way as idiopathic cases. Less commonly, bleeding in DLE may be associated with a circulating anticoagulant.

Renal failure

The anaemia of renal failure is that discussed under 'anaemia of chronic disorders'. In addition, loss of erythropoietin normally

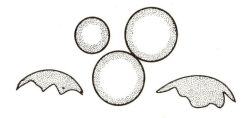

Red blood cells in uraemia

Fig. 19.3 Red cells in uraemia.

produced by the kidney, may contribute to the severe anaemia that may occur in uraemia.

The blood film in uraemia may show burr cells or helmet cells of the type illustrated in Fig. 19.3.

Hypersegmented neutrophils may be present.

Uraemic patients may develop a bleeding tendency other than that due to disseminated intravascular coagulation. This bleeding tendency may be associated with only moderate reduction of platelet numbers but with a long bleeding time. Platelet release phenomena are abnormal and these include defects of platelet adhesiveness, aggregation and platelet factor 3 release. These abnormalities are corrected after haemodialysis and this suggests the presence on the platelets of a retained metabolite derived from plasma interfering with their function.

Thyroid disease

Apart from the strong association of thyroid disease with pernicious anaemia—10 per cent of myxoedema patients and 1 per cent of thyrotoxic patients have pernicious anaemia, disease of the thyroid has an important effect on haemopoiesis. Red cell mass is increased in thyrotoxic patients (overactive thyroid) and decreased in myxoedematous patients (underactive thyroid).

Mild anaemia may sometimes be found in myxoedema but almost all patients show a variable degree of macrocytosis that returns to normal within a few months of replacement therapy. In some the MCV may be very high but even where the MCV is within the normal range it declines significantly when the patient becomes euthyroid. This macrocytosis is not due to vitamin B_{12} deficiency (unless pernicious anaemia is associated) and the marrow is normoblastic.

In addition, about one third of the patients with myxoedema have

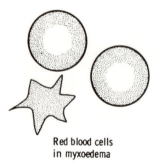

Red blood cells
in myxoedema

Fig. 19.4 Crenated red cells in myxoedema.

occasional irregularly-crenated red cells as illustrated in Fig. 19.4.

Some patients with hyperthyroidism have abnormally small red cells which become normocytic only after they become euthyroid.

Alcoholism

Excess chronic alcohol consumption generally produces changes in the blood. The commonest seen in over 80 per cent of alcoholics is macrocytosis. More severe and more acute alcoholic intoxication in addition to macrocytosis may produce changes in the marrow of the same kind that is seen with other marrow toxins such as chloramphenicol. These are megaloblastic changes, pathological ringed sideroblasts and vacuolation in haemopoietic precursor cells. These toxic effects disappear within 6-10 days of alcohol withdrawal. During the phase of excess alcohol intake, there is suppression of haemopoiesis with a low reticulocyte count, a falling platelet count and a high serum iron level. Recovery following alcohol withdrawal is accompanied by a fall in the serum iron level and a reticulocytosis. In the longer term red cell size will become normal if abstention from alcohol is maintained.

Alcohol also affects other tissues such as the liver, pancreas, and gastrointestinal tract and its mode of action is not known. It is *not* through the folate co-enzymes since in the absence of dietary deficiency of folate, liver, red cell and serum folate levels are unaffected.

In about one third of chronic alcoholics in the United Kingdom, megaloblastic anaemia due to folic-acid deficiency appears. This is due to associated dietary inadequacy. It occurs in those not taking normal meals and in those drinking spirits and wine which do not supply much folate. It is much less frequent in beer drinkers since this contains significant amounts of folic acid. This anaemia responds to oral folate therapy; the macrocytosis of chronic alcoholism is unaffected by folate treatment.

Liver disease

Anaemia is often that encountered in 'anaemia of chronic disorders'. Distinctive features particularly in obstructive jaundice are the presence of target cells. The presence of an enlarged spleen may sometimes produce neutropenia and/or thrombocytopenia due to excessive removal of these cells by the spleen (hypersplenism).

Abnormal bleeding in liver disease (apart from that due to varices) may result from a failure of synthesis of coagulation factors. In obstructive jaundice vitamin K is not absorbed, and vitamin K dependent factors are not synthesized. This defect is easily corrected

Table 19.1 The diagnosis of malaria in blood films

Stage of Parasite	P. falciparum	P. vivax	P. malariae	P. ovale
Young trophozoites (ring form)	Round rings $1/8$–$1/2$ RBC diameter. Cytoplasmic ring may be fine or thick and irregular. Multiple rings and Accolé forms are common. Rings are often the only form to be seen in the peripheral blood. Maurer's clefts in red cell.	Oval rings $1/5$ RBC diameter. One side of ring broader than opposite side. Small reddish dot on fine side of ring (chromatin dot). Rare to find two chromatin dots or more than one ring per cell. RBC normal size.	Oval rings $1/3$–$1/2$ RBC diameter. Similar to vivax ring but with cytoplasmic circle thicker.	Oval rings $1/3$ RBC diameter. Cytoplasmic ring thicker than vivax.
Large trophozoite	Not usually to be seen in peripheral blood films.	Parasite contains golden brown pigment. Arreoloid in form $3/4$ of red cell filled. Red cell enlarged and contains reddish dots (Schuffner's dots).	Round or band shaped parasite with black or brown pigment. Red cell not enlarged.	Round parasite with brown grains of pigment. Red cell may be oval and crenated and containing James's dots.
Mature schizont	Not usually to be seen in peripheral blood films.	Parasite completely filling very large red cell 16–24 small round merozoites with chromatin dots irregularly distributed over parasite area.	Large parasite completely filling normal sized red cell. 6–12 merozoites probably in the form of a rosette.	Parasite does not entirely fill the oval enlarged crenated stippled red cell.
Gametocytes	Crescent shape.	Thick blue ring with central chromatin dot enlarged red cell filled.	Round parasite filling normal sized red cell.	Round parasite.
Geographical Distribution	Tropics and subtropics. Most cases in temperate zones involve travellers from Africa.	More common in temperate than tropical regions; often in travellers from India and Pakistan.	Common in tropical Africa, Burma, Ceylon and India.	Least common of four species occurs mostly in tropical West Africa and Ethiopia.

by vitamin K injections. The characteristic laboratory finding is a very prolonged prothrombin time, with moderate prolongation of the Kaolin-cephalin time. In severe liver failure there is a depletion of all liver-produced factors: vitamin K-dependent factors, factor V, fibrinogen and plasma proteinase inhibitors. In addition, as the liver fails to clear activated clotting factors, disseminated intravascular clotting may supervene, often accompanied by very high levels of factor VIII. The bleeding is extremely difficult to control. Fresh whole blood and fresh plasma are used.

Haemochromatosis
This is a familial disease in which there is excessive storage of iron in the body due to excessive absorption from the gut. As a result there is damage to and fibrosis of the liver, pancreas and other organs. The blood count is essentially normal, the serum iron is high with saturation of the transferrin. Marrow shows reticulum cells heavily loaded with iron. Treatment is by regular venesection.

Felty's syndrome
Patients with this syndrome have rheumatoid arthritis, a large spleen and severe neutropenia. The platelets may be reduced. Because of the severe neutropenia patients suffer severe and frequent infections. Some patients improve on splenectomy.

Malaria
Air travel has made malaria a relatively common disorder in those coming from endemic areas. Table 19.1 sets out the morphological criteria in diagnosis as well as the geographical distribution of different types.

Reference
Israels M C G, Delamore I W 1972 Haematological aspects of systemic disease. Clinics in Haematology. Saunders, London.

20

Pregnancy and the blood

Physiology   Haemolytic disease of the newborn
Iron   Haemostasis
Folate

Physiological adjustments. Human gestation lasts for 40 weeks and during this period there are considerable changes in the blood as compared to the non-pregnant state. The plasma volume starts to increase early in pregnancy and reaches a maximum after the 30th week when the increase is approximately 1000 ml. There is a smaller increase in red cell volume of about 300 ml. As a result the concentration of haemoglobin falls (Fig. 20.1) till about 30 weeks when it increases again.

There is a significant increase in the MCV by an average of 4 fl but this can be as high as 20 fl in some women. It returns to pre-pregnancy values postpartum.

There is a small increase in the white cell count due to increased numbers of neutrophils, and about one in five pregnant women have total white cell counts greater than 10 000/μl. Metamyelocytes normally appear in the blood in pregnancy.

There is a decrease in platelets from a mean of 305 000/μl at 11–15 weeks to 268 000/μl in the last 4 weeks of pregnancy. There is probably increased platelet adhesiveness. Following delivery there is a rise in platelet numbers.

The importance of iron

Iron requirements increase considerably in pregnancy. This increased iron requirement arises from:

Normal iron losses (1 mg/day for 40 weeks)	280 mg
Expansion of red cell mass in pregnancy	570 mg
Iron transferred to the fetus	200–370 mg
Iron content of placenta and cord	30–170 mg
Blood loss in delivery	100–250 mg
Lactation for six months	100–180 mg

At the same time there is no menstrual blood loss for 15 months and this conserves between 240–480 mg of iron. Not all the additional iron needed in pregnancy is lost to the mother since the iron in the increased red cell mass is retained. Overall, during pregnancy between 700–1400 mg of additional iron must be found. The increased need for iron occurs in the latter two thirds of pregnancy. As a physiological response to increased iron need the same improvement in intestinal absorption of dietary iron occurs in pregnancy as in iron-deficiency anaemia so that about 4 mg is absorbed daily as opposed to 1–1½ mg. At the same time the transferrin concentration increases as it does in uncomplicated iron deficiency. In practice very few women are able to meet the iron needs of pregnancy without taking additional iron. Iron-

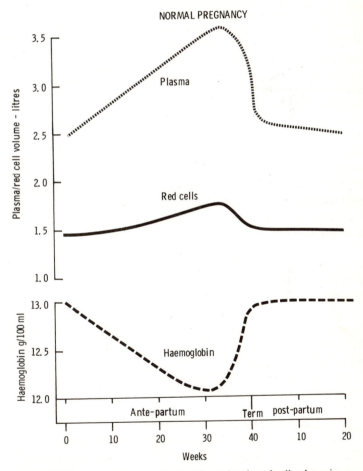

Fig. 20.1 The greater increase in plasma volume than in red cell volume in pregnancy leads to a decline in haemoglobin concentration due to dilution. This trend is reversed before term.

deficiency anaemia is the commonest and most important form of anaemia in pregnancy.

The normal range of haemoglobin concentration at the 30th week of pregnancy in women who have received parenteral iron is from 10.0 to 14.5 g/100 ml. Nevertheless haemodilution is so variable that some patients may have evidence of iron deficiency when the haemoglobin is greater than 11.0 g/100 ml. A better guide to the diagnosis of iron deficiency in pregnancy is the MCV and the MCH. If these two are abnormally low and the patient has not got thalassaemia trait, the woman should be regarded as having iron-deficiency anaemia and treated accordingly. Prophylactic iron is usually given throughout pregnancy. A single tablet containing 30 mg elemental iron taken daily, is adequate. In the absence of regular prophylactic iron about one third of women taking an adequate mixed diet show evidence of iron-deficiency anaemia in the second half of pregnancy. Under less satisfactory nutritional circumstances almost all pregnant women will become iron deficient. Anaemia is more frequent in women having their third or fourth child particularly if the periods between pregnancies were rather short.

Folic acid in pregnancy

Folate co-enzymes are needed for the synthesis of new purines and pyrimidines. These are used to make the nucleic acids of new cells. With rapid growth of the uterus, placenta and fetus there is a greatly increased requirement for folic acid in pregnancy.

To meet the folate needs of the vast majority of pregnant women on mixed diets an additional 200 μg folate has to be supplied each day. This figure is based on studies of red cell folate concentrations throughout pregnancy. The red cell folate level continued to decline throughout pregnancy when 50 μg folate was given daily; the mean red cell folate after the 20th week was maintained on 100 μg folate daily but many individual patients still showed falling folate levels, and on 200 μg folate daily almost all women maintained or increased their red cell folate levels. This level of folate largely prevents the development of megaloblastic marrow changes.

If folate deficiency develops, a megaloblastic anaemia may appear. In adequately nourished women this is usually a very mild 'anaemia' in 1 to 2 per cent of women, which disappears without treatment after the birth of the child. Severe megaloblastic anaemia in pregnancy in western countries is relatively unusual. In badly nourished populations severe anaemia in pregnancy is commonplace. While most anaemias in pregnancy are due to iron deficiency, in malnourished populations megaloblastic anaemia is common.

The earliest evidence of a megaloblastic process is a rising MCV in the blood count. In pregnancy, however, this is often a physiological change but may be of greater pathological significance when accompanied by anaemia. The blood film may show occasional macrocytes or the red cells may be uniformly increased in size. There may be some neutrophils with five or six lobes to the nucleus (up to 3 per cent of five-lobed forms are seen normally). The only reliable means of diagnosing early megaloblastic change in pregnancy is by marrow aspiration. In the absence of folate supplements such changes are found in no less than 25 per cent of women in late pregnancy.

If the changes progress, a more typical megaloblastic picture emerges (Ch. 12). Diagnosis is usually made either in the last few weeks of pregnancy or after the birth of the child (puerperium).

Diagnosis often is complicated by simultaneous iron deficiency, and this may make recognition of the marrow changes more difficult.

Folate deficiency in pregnancy not only increases the risk for the mother but also adversely affects the infant. There is a very high frequency of premature births, that is of infants born several weeks before full term. Such infants are small, often well below 2·27 kg (five pounds). This in turn is the result of an abnormally small placenta. Prematurity and low birth weight infants are prevented by folate supplementation in pregnancy.

Megaloblastic anaemia is more frequent where in addition to pregnancy there is some further extra folate requirement. This is the case in twin pregnancy where megaloblastic anaemia is ten times more likely than in a woman carrying a single child. Severe megaloblastic anaemia is also more likely if there is an associated haemolytic anaemia. This is commonly so in West Africa where one third of the indigenous population carry a gene for either sickle cell haemoglobin or haemoglobin C and where malaria infestation (which also produces haemolysis) is common. Pregnancy in epileptic patients taking anticonvulsant drugs, which of themselves are associated with folate deficiency, often leads to a megaloblastic anaemia. Where there is an additional factor leading to folate deficiency megaloblastic anaemia occurs earlier even at the 20–25th week of pregnancy.

Laboratory tests are of little value in diagnosis of folate deficiency in pregnancy. Serum folate falls in normal pregnancy reaching the lowest level at term and is often as low in normoblastic as in megaloblastic patients. The red cell folate is abnormally low in only half the patients with megaloblastic marrows. This is because change in red cell folate is relatively slow as a new red cell population produced by the folate-deficient marrow is required to replace the older red cells before really low folate levels are reached. Because of changes in intestinal absorption and renal function in pregnancy, tests like 'Figlu excretion' are often normal despite severe folate deficiency.

The serum vitamin B_{12} level normally falls in pregnancy and in about one in 20 women the level may be below 170 pg/ml. The explanation for this is that there is preferential transfer of vitamin B_{12} taken in from the diet to the fetus at the expense of maintaining the level in the plasma. A healthy women has about 3000 μg of vitamin B_{12}; the new born infant only about 50 μg. Thus pregnancy of itself is of minor importance in reducing maternal vitamin B_{12} stores and pregnancy is never a cause of vitamin B_{12} deficiency.

Prediction and management of haemolytic disease of the newborn during pregnancy

During labour, in the course of any obstetric manipulations, or during a miscarriage or even in the absence of these factors, some haemorrhage may occur at the attachment of the placenta to the uterine wall resulting in a small amount of fetal blood reaching the mother's circulation. The quantity is very small, often less than 0·1 ml. Nevertheless, if the fetal red blood cells contain antigens lacking in the mother's red cells, the fetal cells may stimulate the mother to produce antibodies. In the vast majority of cases the fetus is Rhesus positive (inherited from a Rh positive father), and the mother Rhesus negative, so that anti-Rh antibodies are produced. Should the fetus in the next pregnancy also be Rhesus positive, maternal antibody crossing the placenta may produce a haemolytic anaemia in the infant *in utero*. In 2 per cent of cases, haemolytic disease of the newborn is due to antibodies other than Rhesus. The usual antibody is anti-D, thereafter other Rhesus antibodies and more rarely anti-K and anti-Fy[a]. The management of the newborn is discussed in Chapter 21.

Antenatal testing during pregnancy. When a pregnant women is seen for the first time a blood sample is sent for ABO and Rhesus grouping and the serum is tested against a red cell panel containing all the important major blood group antigens. Both enzyme and antiglobulin methods are used in screening the serum for antibodies. 85 per cent of women are Rhesus positive and the serum should not contain any abnormal antibodies. It is desirable but not essential that this group of women be screened again at 34 weeks of pregnancy.

It is not usual to screen routinely for immune anti-A or anti-B in group O women since haemolytic disease of the newborn due to anti-A (or anti-B) although common, never requires clinical intervention during pregnancy and the presence of immune anti-A in sera is far more common than the corresponding disease due to anti-A. Where however, there is a previous history of ABO haemolytic disease it is as well to determine whether the haemolysin in mother's blood is IgG (which can cross the placenta) or IgM (which cannot). Dithiothreitol added to serum destroys IgM leaving IgG to be titred separately. A titre above 1 in 64 may be significant.

Rhesus negative women without antibodies are retested at the 24th, 30th and 36th week of pregnancy. After birth of a D-positive infant these women must be given anti-D to prevent sensitization. If there is a history of affected infants and no antibodies are found, maternal serum should be tested against the father's cells to detect rare or private antigens.

When an antibody is found. If an antibody is discovered on testing the serum, its specificity is determined by testing the serum against a panel of red cells of known genotype. Cold antibodies are quite common and because they are generally of IgM type which do not cross the placenta, and because they are of a low thermal amplitude, they are rarely of obstetric importance. The commonest of these are Lewis antibodies. All other antibodies are potentially important and the commonest are Rhesus antibodies. The titre of the antibody is determined using an antiglobulin technique and if possible the amount of antibody in terms of $\mu g/ml$ measured usually indirectly by obtaining the titre on an autoanalyzer where the equivalent value in μg of antibody is known.

Not all Rhesus negative women carrying a Rh-positive infant become sensitized even in the absence of prophylactic anti-D in the puerperium. In 1 in 10 matings among Caucasians the mother will be Rh-negative and fetus Rh-positive. Sensitization does not occur as a result of a first pregnancy unless the mother has had a previous abortion or received an injection or transfusion of blood. Nevertheless, about 0·8 per cent of Rh negative women get Rh antibodies at the end of the first pregnancy, presumably due to sensitization during pregnancy. Usually when sensitization occurs anti-Rh appears six months after delivery in 6–8 per cent women. Towards the end of the second 'Rh-positive' pregnancy, antibody appears in 17 per cent of Rh negative women. There is only a small increase in those becoming sensitized in subsequent pregnancies. Thus the majority of Rh negative women bearing Rh positive babies do not develop Rhesus antibodies.

Rhesus immunization is less likely if there is ABO incompatability between mother and fetus because such fetal cells reaching the mother's circulation will be cleared and destroyed, and are therefore less capable of stimulating Rh antibodies.

Of the Rhesus antibodies formed, 93 per cent are anti-D or anti-C+D, and 6 per cent anti-c, anti-E or anti-C+e. The D antigen is obviously the most potent antigen within the Rh system.

Assessment of severity of disease in the fetus

Once antibodies that may cause haemolytic disease of the newborn are found, management is directed to safeguarding the fetus. Decision may be required whether to allow pregnancy to go to term, or because about half the infants who die *in utero* do so in the last few weeks, whether to induce labour early? Is intrauterine transfusion to the fetus indicated and what advice about the outcome can one give to the mother?

History in earlier pregnancies. If a mother has had an infant only mildly affected with haemolytic disease of the newborn, other siblings are also likely to be only mildly affected. A severely affected infant is likely to be followed by other equally or more severely affected ones.

The husband's genotype. When an antibody is discovered the father should be genotyped. If he is heterozygous there is a 50 per cent chance that the infant is unaffected. This may be suggested by failure of the mother's antibody titre to rise during pregnancy. The father's genotype however only gives a probability that he is heterozygous since the 'd' antigen cannot be detected. Genotype of other children will help to reduce the degree of uncertainty. The father's genotype of course, is needed for genetic counselling in relation to the outcome of future pregnancies. If the father is homozygous all infants will be affected.

The antibody titre. The antibody should be titrated at two-weekly intervals throughout pregnancy using an antiglobulin technique. Low titre antibodies (less than 1 in 32) are likely to be associated with mildly affected infants; high titres (more than 1 in 256 at 34 weeks) with severely affected infants. An antibody titre by the antiglobulin method of 1 in 32 (equivalent to $1 \cdot 0$ μg/ml antibody) is an indication for early amniocentesis at about 22–26 weeks.

Amniocentesis. The inner lining of the womb during pregnancy is the amniotic membrane and the fetus grows inside this bag surrounded by a clear straw coloured fluid secreted by the lining cells of the amnion called amniotic fluid. If the Rhesus antibody crossing the placenta is producing a haemolytic anaemia *in utero* there will be increased bile pigment production from the increased destruction of fetal red blood cells and hence an increased bilirubin level in the amniotic fluid. The process of inserting a needle straight through the mother's abdominal wall and wall of the uterus into the amniotic space and drawing off a few ml of amniotic fluid, is called amniocentesis. The placenta must be localized so that the needle does not enter this area but nevertheless puncture of a fetal vessel with bleeding into the amniotic fluid can occur. The colour of the amniotic fluid is noted, and any blood is removed by careful centrifugation. When a blood-stained sample of liquor is obtained a Kleihauer test should be carried out to see if the cells are maternal or fetal. If they are fetal cells they should be grouped (are they Rh positive?) and do they give a positive direct antiglobulin test confirming that the fetus is affected. Particles and vernix which cover the fetus are removed by filtering the fluid through a Hemmings filter. The sample is protected from light and its absorption spectrum is recorded in a continuous reading spectro-photometer between 320 to 600 nanometers. In an uncontaminated liquor a direct reading of bilirubin is obtained by the absorption at 450 nm. The presence of altered blood pigments is shown in the absorption spectrum. Where this is the case other means are used to assess bilirubin content.

When a woman is already immunized the first sample for amniocentesis should be taken between 22 to 26 weeks of pregnancy depending on assessment of severity of the disease. Thereafter it should be repeated at 30 and 34–35 weeks.

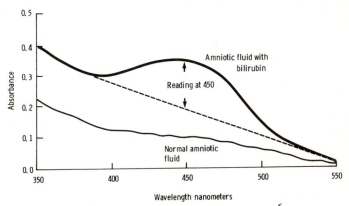

Fig. 20.2 The absorption spectrum of liquor amnii containing bilirubin.

The hump in the absorption spectrum at 450 nm due to bilirubin is shown in Figure 20.2. The absorption at 450 is read and plotted on a chart comparing absorption at various periods of pregnancy (Fig. 20.3). The change in the value at 450 nm with the advance of pregnancy is of importance. In normal pregnancy this value falls as term approaches. A rising value with successive samples of amniotic fluid indicates increasing bilirubin content. Liley has indicated three zones (Fig. 20.3) which roughly correlate with prognosis. Bilirubin values in the lower zone suggest a Rh negative infant, an unaffected Rh positive child or a very mildly affected child. The intermediate area indicates haemolytic disease of intermediate severity and values in the upper zone indicate severely affected infants who might die *in utero*.

Altered haemoglobin due to bleeding from a previous amino-centesis provides additional difficulty since those pigments absorb

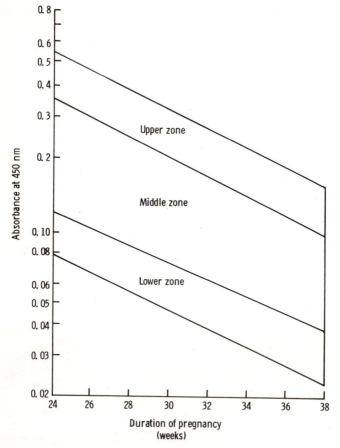

Fig. 20.3 Interpretation of results of amniocentesis. A result in the lower zone suggests an unaffected child or very mildly affected child, a result in the intermediate zone haemolytic disease of intermediate severity and values in the upper zone severely affected infants.

strongly at 410 nm. In order to obtain bilirubin values under these circumstances extinctions are read at 454, 490, 520 and 574nm and E 454–574 and E 490–520 estimated. These values are plotted and interpreted in the same way as the E 450 (Fig. 20.4).

Amniocentesis should be performed only after the subject has emptied her bladder since the mother's urine will produce a strange absorption spectrum. Ascitic fluid, if present, may also be misleading. During an intrauterine transfusion a radio opaque substance may be injected into the infants peritoneal cavity and this, appearing in the liquor, may present difficulties in obtaining reliable readings in subsequent amniocentesis. Amniocentesis in an unsensitized mother does present the risk of sensitization as fetal cells may appear in the mother's blood.

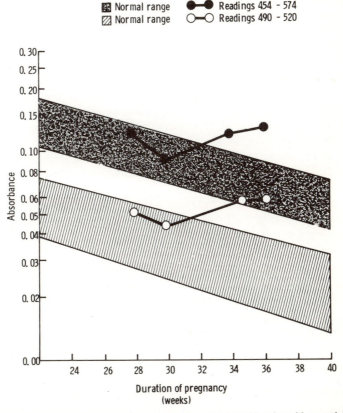

Fig. 20.4 Plotting of results with liquor amnii contaminated by altered haemoglobin. Absorptions results derived from 454 minus 574 and 490 minus 520 are plotted. The points indicate the rising bilirubin level with an affected fetus.

Management of haemolytic disease of the newborn during pregnancy. A rising maternal antibody titre, a history of severely affected infants or stillbirth and a rising bilirubin level on amniocentesis or an initial elevated value all indicate the need for active measures. It is generally agreed that premature delivery of the infant at about 36 weeks is desirable. Earlier induction carries an unacceptably high neonatal mortality. To avoid stillbirth before the fetus is old enough to be delivered with a reasonable chance of survival it is necessary to transfuse the fetus with Rh-negative blood which will not be destroyed by the antibody. These transfusions are carried out by passing a cannula into the fetus's abdominal cavity and running in between 60–120 ml fresh Rhesus negative blood as packed cells. This may be done initially at twenty-four weeks and if necessary repeated at two weekly intervals till thirty-five weeks when the infant can be delivered.

Prevention of Rhesus sensitization

Sensitization of an Rh-negative woman by blood cells entering the mother's circulation from the fetus can be prevented if she is given 100 μg anti-D within three days of delivery. The anti-D coats the Rhesus-positive cells, and by causing their rapid clearance from the circulation prevents them from initiating an immune response. The mechanism of 'immunosuppression' is related to removal of the fetal cells and can be brought about by antibodies other than anti-D such, as anti-K in the case of D positive Kell-positive fetal cells or by ABO incompatability.

All Rhesus negative women with a Rhesus positive infant must be given anti-D, as should such women after abortion or unsensitized women after amniocentesis or obstetric manipulation such as turning the fetus from breech to cephalic position (version).

Fetal cells can be demonstrated in the maternal circulation by treating the blood film with a pH 3·3 buffer when HbA is denatured but HbF remains largely unchanged. Fetal cells containing HbF can then be stained whereas the maternal cells show as ghosts. This technique makes it possible to obtain a rough assessment of the size of the bleed since more anti-D may be needed for the unusual situation when five or more ml of fetal blood has crossed to the mother.

On rare occasions a large amount of Rh positive cells is transfused to a Rh negative subject. Sensitization to the antigen can be prevented if enough anti-D for example 1000 μg every 24 hours is given. A large volume of Rh positive cells such as a unit of blood may not be cleared from the circulation for several days.

Haemostasis in pregnancy

Haemostasis undergoes a number of changes in pregnancy which are directed to ensuring rapid and effective control of bleeding following separation of the placenta. These changes become detectable early in the second trimester and consist of a steady rise in fibrinogen concentration up to $6.0 \, g/l$ and increased levels of factors VII, VIII and X. The plasminogen concentration is also increased. At the same time there is a reduced fibrinolytic capacity due to markedly decreased plasminogen activator levels and increased levels of inhibitors of the fibrinolytic system.

Immediately after the birth of the infant the plasminogen activator levels rise to normal. Coagulation factors return to pre-pregnancy values.

Thrombo-embolism in pregnancy. The hypercoagulable state present in pregnancy is associated with an increased frequency of deep vein thrombosis and pulmonary embolism. There is a particularly high risk of these complications in the puerperium. Pregnant women with these complications or with a history of thrombo-embolism in a previous pregnancy or apart from pregnancy, should be treated with anticoagulants (Ch. 22). The oral anticoagulant drugs readily cross the placenta and depress the activity of the vitamin K-dependent factors in the fetus. In addition they may produce congenital malformation if given in the early weeks of pregnancy. For these reasons oral anticoagulants are not given in early pregnancy (first trimester) and are withdrawn about four weeks before term. Heparin is used instead over these periods either 30–40 000 units per day i.v. by continuous infusion or 5–10 000 units subcutaneously, twice daily.

Disseminated intravascular coagulation in pregnancy. Several important obstetric complications act as the trigger setting off DIC. These are accidental haemorrhage, retained dead fetus, amniotic fluid embolism, septic abortion, pre-eclampsia and eclampsia.

Concealed accidental haemorrhage or premature separation of the placenta is accompanied by shock. Even in the absence of overt bleeding, abnormal laboratory tests indicative of DIC are often present. With delivery of the fetus and treatment of shock, the coagulation abnormalities correct themselves. Prompt replacement of the blood volume is particularly important; replacement therapy with fresh frozen plasma and platelet concentrates is occasionally required.

Retention of a dead fetus for several weeks may be accompanied by a gradual fall in fibrinogen, factor VIII and platelets with a rise in fibrin degradation products. DIC under these circumstances is probably due to the release of thromboplastic substances from the intrauterine contents. If evidence of defective haemostasis is present heparin (20000–30000 iu intravenously for 24–48 hours) is given, followed by measures to evacuate the uterus.

Amniotic fluid embolism may occur during or after labour or Caesarian section, with an acute onset of shock, respiratory distress, and cyanosis. Severe bleeding from the uterus and other sites follows.

The amniotic fluid directly activates factor X and this in turn converts prothrombin to thrombin. The right heart strain due to pulmonary embolism, makes transfusion difficult and dangerous for the patient. Slow and carefully controlled infusions of blood and fresh frozen plasma, as well as heparin (1000 iu per hour) are given.

DIC is sometimes associated with intrauterine infections, and abortion induced with hypertonic solutions. Low-grade DIC is present in pre-eclampsia and eclampsia and may be associated with fibrin deposition in maternal vessels in the placenta, liver and kidney.

References

Hathaway W E, Bonnar J 1978 Perinatal coagulation. Grune & Stratton, New York

Mollison P L 1979 Blood transfusion in clinical medicine, 6th ed. Blackwell, Oxford

21

Some haematological problems in infancy

Haemolytic disease of the newborn
Transplacental haemorrhage
Neonatal thrombocytopenia

Haemostasis in the newborn
Haemolytic uraemic syndrome
Vitamin E deficiency

Haemolytic disease of the newborn *(Erythroblastosis fetalis)*
This disorder is due to maternal antibodies crossing the placenta and reacting with the red blood cells of the fetus. The survival of these fetal red cells is thus shortened in the same way as are the red cells in an adult with autoimmune haemolytic anaemia.

In the vast majority of affected infants, *erythroblastosis fetalis* is due to a maternal IgG immunoglobin of Rhesus specificity crossing the placenta; in about 2 per cent of cases it is due to other blood group antibodies. Antibodies in the ABO system are even more common as causes of mild haemolytic disease of the newborn than Rhesus antibodies, but ABO incompatibility is rarely of sufficient severity to need clinical intervention.

Antenatal management is discussed in the chapter on 'Pregnancy and the blood'. This section is concerned with the events in the newborn. With the exception of a mother having a baby without any antenatal care, the likelihood of a baby having haemolytic disease as well as the probable severity of the disease will be known both from history of earlier pregnancies and from findings in the mother's serum and amniotic fluid. ABO incompatibility is generally diagnosed after birth since routine antenatal screening is not warranted.

Haemolytic disease due to anti-Rh
One in 200 infants is affected by Rhesus sensitization. The more severely affected infants die *in utero* (unless treated with intrauterine transfusion) and this affects 10–20 per cent of all cases. Such infants may be oedematous and pale, and the placenta is also oedematous. The condition is called *hydrops fetalis*. The remaining infants are less severely affected and develop jaundice after birth. The mildest cases merely become anaemic after the second week of life.

Where haemolytic disease is suspected a specimen of blood should be taken with a syringe from the cord before the placenta is delivered.

A blood count, bilirubin estimation, a direct antiglobulin test and ABO and Rhesus grouping is carried out as soon as possible. The infant with haemolytic disease may show pallor and enlarged liver and spleen. Jaundice is absent at birth because the bilirubin produced by the fetus *in utero* is largely excreted via the placenta and metabolized by the maternal liver. The liver of the newborn infant generally has a low capacity to conjugate bilirubin, that is, the enzyme glucuronyl-transferase, is poorly developed at birth. For this reason increased red cell destruction rapidly leads to a rise in the plasma levels of unconjugated bilirubin starting in the second 24 hours of life. High levels of unconjugated bilirubin are dangerous in infants because it gives rise to permanent brain damage (kernicterus) 20 mg bilirubin per 100 ml (342 μmol/l) being regarded as the dangerous level.

Laboratory findings. Half the affected infants are anaemic. The blood film shows polychromasia and many normoblasts but the red cells remain normocytic unlike ABO haemolytic disease where spherocytes are a feature. The reticulocyte count is high. The direct antiglobulin test is strongly positive. It is important that the tests be carried out on cord blood, since this gives the most reliable guide as to the severity of the disorder and hence the line of treatment to be followed. Normal cord blood haemoglobin concentration is 13·6 to 19·6 g/100 ml (it is 2–3 g higher from a heel prick after birth) and normal cord blood bilirubin is up to 3 mg/100 ml (51·3 μmol/l).

Decision as to whether to proceed to an exchange transfusion is taken on the basis of previous history of an affected infant, clinical state of the baby, the haemoglobin and bilirubin level. Above 40 per cent of affected infants require no treatment. History of a previously exchanged infant, a cord haemoglobin below 12 g/100 ml and a bilirubin level about 4 mg/100 ml (68·4 μmol/l) are positive indications for exchange. On the other hand a full term infant with a cord haemoglobin above 14 g/100 ml and a bilirubin below 3 mg (51·3 μmol/l) should be watched. After birth a rising bilirubin level and a falling haemoglobin concentration may indicate need for treatment, the prime object being to prevent accumulation of bilirubin which may lead to kernicterus.

Management. The purpose of exchange transfusion is to remove the infant's antibody-coated red cells which will yield more bilirubin and replace them with Rh negative cells. Removal of bilirubin is also achieved and this is the main objective of later exchanges. Ideally fresh Rhesus negative whole blood either in heparin or CPD of the same ABO group as the infant, is used. Partly packed cells may be needed for severely anaemic infants. The blood should be compatible with the mother's serum. Exchange is effected by removing 10–20 ml aliquots of infant's blood, returning the same amount of Rhesus negative blood and using a total of 160–180 ml blood per kg of body weight. Less severely affected anaemic infants may only require a simple transfusion.

Phototherapy, that is exposure of the infant to bright light as in a series of fluorescent tubes, stimulates excretion of bilirubin in the urine. It is used in infants at risk from rising bilirubin levels both before and after exchange transfusion. Phenobarbitone has also been used but is less effective.

Haemolytic disease due to ABO incompatibility

In 20 per cent of pregnancies there is ABO incompatibility between mother and fetus. The commonest combination is an O mother with either a group A or group B fetus and this is the combination giving rise to haemolytic disease. Sera from group O mothers whose infants have ABO haemolytic disease, show immune as compared to naturally-acquired anti-A or anti-B. Naturally acquired anti-A or anti-B is mainly an IgM immunoglobin. Exposure of maternal antiserum to 2-mercaptoethanol or dithiothreitol destroys IgM, the remaining reaction against A or B cells being due to IgG antibodies. These immune antibodies are haemolytic.

Haemolytic disease due to anti-A or less commonly, anti-B, is a mild disorder, rarely requiring active treatment. The reason is that A and B antigens are poorly developed on infant red cells. Secondly IgG anti-A or anti-B crossing the placenta, is partially neutralized by A or B substance free in the fetal plasma. ABO haemolytic disease does not cause intrauterine death and unlike Rh disease, may affect the first baby.

Clinically the appearance of early jaundice may raise the suspicion of haemolytic disease. The haemoglobin level is usually normal but the stained film shows some polychromasia There is a reticulocytosis and increased number of normoblasts. Spherocytosis is usually prominent. The direct antiglobulin test is usually negative or weakly positive. The infants serum may show free antibody against adult red cells.

Management. Infants are treated with phototherapy and bilirubin levels watched. An exchange is indicated if the level of unconjugated bilirubin exceeds 20 mg/100 ml (342 μmol/l). Group O blood is used, preferably washed once in saline and red cells suspended in AB plasma.

Other causes of neonatal jaundice

Rarely other blood disorders may be the cause of jaundice in the first few days of life that must be differentiated from haemolytic disease of the newborn. These include hereditary spherocytosis and glucose-6-phosphate dehydrogenase deficiency. Internal haemorrhage is another cause. Vitamin K medication may also lead to jaundice.

Transplacental and other haemorrhages

Blood loss should always be considered as a possible explanation for anaemia in the newborn. External haemorrhage may be associated with obstetric accidents or placenta praevia. Internal haemorrhage may be associated with jaundice. Large transplacental haemorrhage (50 ml of blood or more) will produce distress in the infant with anaemia and later polychromasia and many normoblasts in the film. Diagnosis rests on demonstrating fetal cells in appropriate numbers in maternal blood. Treatment is by transfusion.

Occasionally twin bleeds occur, one twin being anaemic and the other polycythaemic. In these cases there are anastomoses between the placentae. A haemoglobin difference of greater than 5g/100ml between twins is suggestive that this has occurred.

Bleeding disorders of the newborn

The normal premature and term infant has 'physiological' deficiencies of vitamin K dependent factors (II, VII, IX and X) and contact factors (XI and XII) resulting in prolongation of thrombin and kaolin-cephalin time. Fibrinogen is present in normal adult quantities, although its clotting function is reduced, possibly due to the presence of fetal fibrinogen. Thrombin time is prolonged. Factors V, VIIIC and VIIIRAg are normal. Factor XIII and plasminogen are reduced to about 50 per cent of adult normal. Overall fibrinolytic activity is normal except during the first day of life when it is increased. The physiological inhibitors are normal, except for a reduction in antithrombin III levels. Platelets are normal in number, but fail to aggregate to collagen, ADP, adrenaline and thrombin.

Haemorrhagic disease of the newborn

This is an exaggeration of the normal deficiency of vitamin K dependent factors, sometimes found in breast fed babies. It occurs rarely, if ever, in babies on milk preparations since cows' milk contains four times more vitamin K than human milk. Bleeding starts between the second and the fourth day of life, usually from the umbilical stump or gastrointestinal tract. Laboratory tests disclose a gross prolongation of prothrombin time, corrected by vitamin K_1 (100–500 μg) within six hours of injection. If the bleeding is severe, fresh frozen plasma should be given to cover the period before vitamin K_1 acts.

Infants with chronic diarrhoea, cystic fibrosis or biliary atresia (causing vitamin K *malabsorption*) may develop haemorrhagic disease at a later stage. Severe deficiency of vitamin K dependent factors also occurs in babies born to mothers taking *oral anticoagulants* at the time of delivery. It is therefore important to change from oral anticoagulants to heparin at 36–37 weeks of gestation. Breast milk does not contain significant amounts of oral anticoagulants, and mothers on those drugs should be able to breast feed safely. Infants born to mothers on *anticonvulsant drugs* (phenytoin, barbiturates) may also develop severe haemorrhagic disease. The defect responds promptly to vitamin K_1 and fresh frozen plasma. It can be prevented if vitamin K_1 is given orally to the mother prior to delivery.

Hereditary haemorrhagic defects

Infants with inherited defects of coagulation factors may develop haematomata, bleed after circumcision, have intracranial haemorrhage or bleed from the umbilical stump. Fortunately, the commonest inherited disorder, haemophilia A, rarely causes neonatal bleeding. Massive fatal intracranial haemorrhage has been reported in babies with factor V, X and XI deficiency. Delayed bleeding from the umbilical stump is often found in factor XIII deficiency. Inherited abnormalities of platelet function, such as thrombasthenia or Bernard-Soulier syndrome, may present with severe mucous membrane bleeding and generalized petechiae.

Diagnosis of platelet defects and congenital deficiencies of factors II, VII, IX, X, XI and XII is difficult at birth (see above) and the laboratory results must be confirmed when the child is over 3 months of age. Diagnosis of factor V, VIII, or XIII deficiency, as well as of hypo- or afibrinogenaemia can be made at birth. Babies are treated with the appropriate blood product, observed closely for intracranial haemorrhage and venepunctures avoided whenever possible.

Thrombocytopenia in the neonate

The commonest causes of thrombocytopenia in the neonate are disseminated intravascular clotting, infection and exchange transfusion. Neonates can also develop severe immune thrombocytopenia, as well as thrombocytopenia due to inherited marrow failure or maternal drugs.

Immunologically induced thrombocytopenia can be of two types:

1. Isoimmune, when the mother becomes sensitized to a fetal platelet

antigen, and the resulting antibody destroys platelets in the infant. It is usually due to a platelet specific antigen PL^A, but other platelet or histocompatibility antigens may also be involved.

2. Autoimmune, when maternal antibody produced as part of an autoimmune process (idiopathic thrombocytopenic purpura, disseminated lupus erythematosus) is passively transferred across the placenta and causes thrombocytopenia in the infant.

Typically, the infants platelet count is below 25000/μl and the infant has generalised purpura. Serious bleeding, including CNS haemorrhage, may occur in up to 25 per cent of children affected.

Rarely thrombocytopenia may be due to the absence of megakaryocytes in the bone marrow. It may be associated with bone abnormalities or part of Fanconi's pancytopenia.

Drugs given to the mother, such as tolbutaminde or thiazides, have been associated with neonatal pancytopenia.

Investigation of an infant with thrombocytopenia requires a bone marrow aspirate and serological tests on maternal or infant serum and on paternal platelets. The presence of autoimmune disorder in the mother must be sought. In mildly affected babies with immune thrombocytopenia, no treatment is required and the platelet count returns to normal within 3–4 weeks of delivery. If the infant is bleeding, platelet transfusion or exchange transfusion followed by platelet transfusion are used.

Disseminated intravascular coagulation (DIC)

DIC is the most common cause of bleeding in the sick newborn. It has been well documented in babies born after abruptio placentae or placenta praevia, in hypoxic and acidotic infants, in neonatal bacterial and viral infections, in idiopathic respiratory distress syndrome, haemolytic disease of the newborn, necrotizing enterocolitis and as part of severe liver disease. As in adults, there is a generalized intravascular consumption of clotting factors and platelets. This is frequently associated with widespread microthrombosis leading to ischaemic organ damage. The newborn is particularly prone to DIC because his macrophage-monocytic system is as yet incapable of clearing activated clotting factors and platelets, and his liver is immature and unable to synthesize extra clotting factors to replace those lost during DIC.

The laboratory findings are similar to those in adults: prolonged prothrombin time, kaolin-cephalin and thrombin time, low platelet count, reduced plasma fibrinogen and increased serum FDP concentration. The key to successful treatment of DIC lies in treating the disease that provoked it. Fresh frozen plasma and exchange transfusion with fresh blood may be of benefit. Rarely, if thrombotic manifestations predominate, the infant may require heparinization. One hundred units of heparin per kg of body weight are given every 4 hours.

Haemolytic uraemic syndrome

This is a disease seen in children generally under 2 years of age, presenting with either a chest or gastrointestinal upset, followed 10–12 days later by lethargy, abdominal pain, vomiting, fever and purpura. There is a raised blood pressure and some oedema. Urine has blood and protein.

The blood shows anaemia and reticulocytosis. The film shows polychromasia, red cell fragments and irregularly crenated red cells (burr cells). The platelet count is low and this is part of disseminated intravascular coagulation. There is renal failure with poor output of urine.

Management is concerned with treatment of renal failure. The management of DIC has been discussed. Plasma exchange and administration of fresh frozen plasma have been used with some success.

Vitamin E deficiency

Deficiency of vitamin E (α-tocopherol) can lead to a haemolytic anaemia in premature infants when they reach 6–10 weeks of age. The blood shows some anisocytosis and a reticulocytosis (2–10 per cent). Such red cells are said to be excessively sensitive to hydrogen peroxide which is normally produced in the red cell and this has been developed into a laboratory test for possible vitamin E deficiency. The haemolytic anaemia is said to respond to therapy with vitamin E.

References

Chessels J M, Hardisty R M 1974 Bleeding problems in the newborn infant. In: Spaet T H (ed) Progress in thrombosis and haemostasis. Grune & Stratton, New York, p. 333–361

Hathaway W E, Bonnar J 1978 Perinatal coagulation. Grune & Stratton, New York

22

Thrombosis and its management

Thrombosis is the formation of a thrombus in the lumen of a blood vessel. It results from the breakdown of the normal balance between haemostasis and protective mechanisms, and is initiated by either damage to the vessel wall, by platelet aggregation or by activation of coagulation, alone or in combination.

Arterial thrombosis. Thrombosis in arteries generally follows damage to the endothelium. Platelets adhere to the exposed subintimal layer leading to activation of coagulation and fibrin deposition. The speed and the nature of blood flow (bends, bifurcations etc.) determine whether the platelet-fibrin mass is built up or removed. Arteries other than pulmonary arteries have low fibrinolytic activity and local fibrinolytic mechanisms cannot successfully lyse large fibrin masses.

Venous thrombosis. Factors leading to venous thrombosis are stasis of blood, local activation of coagulation and endothelial damage. Stasis is the most important, and the common stagnant areas are valve pockets of leg veins and venous sinuses in the calf. Muscular action serves to pump blood out of the veins and prolonged immobility in bed or on the operating table leads to venous stasis. Accumulation of activated procoagulants in these areas results in generation of thrombin and this in turn, induces platelet aggregation and formation of fibrin. The fibrin can adhere to venous endothelium and a stable nidus is formed. If there is adequate fibrinolysis and blood flow is restored, the thrombus will not propagate. Otherwise the thrombus will increase in size and may cause clinically overt deep venous thrombosis.

Changes in blood. Hypercoagulability refers to blood changes that may predispose to thrombosis. These occur after trauma, operation, pregnancy, in chronic or acute illness, infection, and in malignant disease. The changes are an increase in concentrations of fibrinogen, factor VIII, factor V, and plasminogen and a decrease in the levels of antithrombin III and fibrinolytic activity. There is an increased platelet count and changed platelet reactivity as detected by increased retention on glass beads and increased aggregability. The changes are shown schematically in Figure 22.1.

Rare familial disorders such as antithrombin III deficiency, dysfibrinogenaemia, or excessively high levels of factor V are associated with an increased frequency of venous thrombosis.

Clinical aspects of venous thrombosis

Venous thrombosis is present in between 20 and 40 per cent of all autopsies. It is impossible to assess the incidence in life as most cases are clinically silent. Most thrombi arise in the calf veins and almost half of these lyse spontaneously after a few days. About 20 per cent become organized, that is, the thrombus is replaced by fibrous tissue, and this may impair the function of valves in the deep veins; another 20 per cent propagate upwards from the calf veins into popliteal, femoral and iliac veins. The thrombi in thigh veins are particularly likely to become detached into the venous circulation and be carried through the right side of the heart to lodge in the lungs.

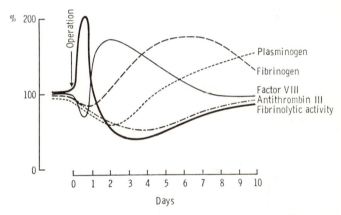

Fig. 22.1 Changes in the blood producing a hypercoagulable state after surgery.

Patients with venous thrombosis often have no symptoms. When effects are produced they may be local, usually a painful or a swollen leg, or due to pulmonary emboli. In the longer term venous thrombosis may lead to a post-thrombotic syndrome. Poor venous return from the leg causes faulty nutrition of tissues with induration, pigmentation and ulceration of the skin. Venous ulcers are usually located on the medial side of the ankle. Ileofemoral thrombosis may give rise to a swollen, painful and heavy leg.

Pulmonary embolism too can be clinically silent or may cause sudden chest pain and haemoptysis with or without shortness of breath. As pulmonary vessels are rich in plasminogen activator, most smaller emboli are quickly lysed. A large embolus interferes with the passage of blood through the affected portion of the lung and this perfusion defect can be demonstrated radiologically. Recurrent embolization may impair the pulmonary circulation and lead to pulmonary hypertension.

Diagnosis of deep venous thrombosis

There may be leg pain, sometimes local venous distension, oedema, tenderness, discoloration and fever. Homan's sign is often positive (pain in the calf on dorsiflexion of the foot). Uncommonly, if the venous return is completely obstructed the entire leg becomes grossly swollen, pale and painful—*phlegmasia alba dolens*. In rare instances the arterial circulation is also impaired, resulting in an oedematous purplish and extremely painful limb—*phlegmasia coerulea dolens*. Help in diagnosis may be sought by:

1. Venography. X-ray following the injection of contrast medium into a foot vein may show a thrombus.
2. Radioactive fibrinogen test. 100 microcuries of I^{125}-labelled fibrinogen is injected i.v. This will label any fibrin laid down at a site of thrombus formation and if this is in the legs the local thrombus can be detected by surface counting. A sudden fall in blood radioactivity in the absence of local thrombus in the leg suggests thrombosis elsewhere in the body. This test is used mostly in detecting calf vein thrombi and noting whether they are lysed or propagated. The test is not reliable in detecting ileofemoral thrombosis.
3. Ultrasound. When a beam of ultrasound reflects from a moving object such as the blood stream, its frequency is altered according to the rate at which the object is moving. This is the Doppler effect. In a patent vein, the velocity of venous flow can be increased by compressing the limb, which causes a change in the signals emitted by the instrument. If there is an obstruction, no change in the signal is elicited by compression. This technique can detect complete obstruction in iliac, femoral and popliteal veins. The test is negative if there is partial occlusion of a vein or if there are large collateral veins. It does not detect thrombi in calf veins.
4. Impedance phlebography. Blood is a good conductor of electricity; an occluded vein in a limb changes the conductivity. This principle is used to detect large occluding thrombi in the thigh veins.

Prophylaxis

The incidence of venous thrombosis is reduced considerably when mechanical devices to prevent venous stasis in the legs or medication to alter blood coagulability, are used.

Elimination of stasis is used in surgical patients. Electrical stimulation of calf muscles during operation, pneumatic compression of the calves via a special 'stocking' during surgery and in the post-operative period, and passive flexion of the foot by motor-driven pedals have been used with success in patients operated on for non-malignant conditions.

There is a significant reduction in the incidence of venous thrombosis and pulmonary embolism if patients are anticoagulated with warfarin at the time of operation. However, due to a greater risk of wound haematomata and post-operative bleeding oral anticoagulants have not been widely adopted. Low dose subcutaneous heparin (5000 iu given 2–3 times daily starting two hours before surgery and continued for 7–14 days) has proved to be effective in preventing venous thrombosis after surgery. It has proved less satisfactory in patients with fractured neck of femur or in patients undergoing operations on the lower limbs. Infusion of low MW Dextran has been used as well.

Management of deep venous thrombosis

General measures. The patient should be confined to bed with the foot of the bed elevated by 15–20 cm and with an elastic bandage applied firmly to below the groin. Regular exercises should be performed, and the patient mobilized as soon as the acute symptoms have disappeared. Analgesics and local heat may help to relieve the pain.

Specific treatment. This consists of anticoagulation, thrombolysis or defibrination. Anticoagulant drugs are commonly used and they prevent further deposition of fibrin and growth of the thrombus, but the treatment does not remove the thrombus. The natural fibrinolytic mechanism may be capable of lysing it once its growth has stopped. Treatment is usually started with 5000 iu of heparin intravenously and continued with 25 iu/kg bodyweight/hour, by intravenous drip or continuous infusion. The duration of heparin treatment depends on the site and extent of thrombosis. For calf-vein thrombosis it is usually given for three days in conjunction with warfarin which is then continued. In ileofemoral thrombosis 7–14 days heparin is followed by warfarin for six weeks to six months depending on the extent of thrombosis and on the presence of post-thrombotic sequelae.

In some cases of acute massive thrombosis, thrombolytic agents, such as streptokinase may be used. Streptokinase treatment is given for 72 hours followed by heparin and long term oral anticoagulants.

Encouraging results have been reported with a purified fraction of the Malayan pit viper venom, Ancrod or Arvin. Ancrod prevents propagation of a thrombus by defibrinating blood.

A small proportion of patients may require surgery such as ligation of the inferior vena cava or the femoral vein, if anticoagulants fail to prevent pulmonary emboli or if anticoagulant therapy is contra-indicated. Rarely surgery may be needed to remove a thrombus if the viability of a leg is in doubt.

Treatment of venous thrombosis must continue after the acute episode has been dealt with. The patient should be advised to take regular exercise and avoid long periods in a sitting position. Elastic stockings or bandages may be of help if oedema persists. The foot of the bed should be elevated until oedema disappears.

Anticoagulation in management of pulmonary embolism. In suspected pulmonary embolism 10 000 iu of heparin is given intravenously at once. Many patients with massive pulmonary embolism die within the first hour and it is often difficult to distinguish between pulmonary embolism, acute myocardial infarction and dissecting aortic aneurysm. If the patient survives, pulmonary angiography is performed and if more than 75 per cent of the vasculature of the lung is occluded surgical removal of the embolus should be carried out. Heparin is given for two weeks after embolectomy and patients are then treated with warfarin for six months.

Patients with smaller pulmonary occlusions are treated by heparin or streptokinase. Streptokinase causes significantly faster lysis of emboli than heparin during the first 24 hours, but after a week there is no difference between the two methods of treatment. A relatively high dose of heparin is needed in the first 24 or 48 hours after a massive embolus (80 000–120 000 iu) and laboratory control is required. Heparin should be continued for up to two weeks, and warfarin then give for six months.

In recurrent pulmonary embolism, anticoagulant treatment must be maintained for long periods of time.

Oral anticoagulants

Mechanism of action and metabolism. Oral anticoagulants are vitamin K antagonists and are either derivatives of coumarin or indanedione compounds. The site of their action is the microsomes of liver cells where they interfere with a later stage of completion of vitamin K-dependent coagulation factors (prothrombin, factor VII, IX and X) and so reduce their concentration in blood. Prothrombin synthesized in the absence of vitamin K does not contain any γ-carboxyglutamic acids necessary for the binding of calcium and is therefore incapable of participating in the coagulation of blood. As shown in Figure 22.2 after warfarin is given, the rate of disappearance of the clotting factors depends on their plasma half life, factor VII falling to very low levels after 24 hours and prothrombin only to half its initial level after three days. The patient is anticoagulated only when the levels of all vitamin K-dependent factors are reduced. For the first 48 to 72 hours after the first dose of warfarin the patient is not protected from thrombosis.

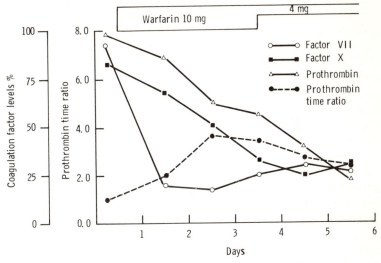

Fig. 22.2 Effect of warfarin on vitamin K-dependent coagulation factors and on the prothrombin time ratio.

Smooth control of anticoagulation is achieved more easily with slowly metabolized drugs (Table 22.1). Warfarin is the most commonly used drug of this group and further discussion will refer mainly to this preparation. Warfarin is almost completely absorbed from the gut and about 97 per cent of the drug in plasma is bound to

Table 22.1 Oral anticoagulants

Proper name	Proprietory name	Gastrointestinal absorption	Plasma half-life hours
Warfarin sodium	Marevan Coumadin	rapid-complete	17–46
Phenindione	Dindevan	rapid-complete	5
Nicoumalone	Sinthrome	rapid-complete	8

albumin. Only the free drug in plasma is effective at the receptor sites. Warfarin is metabolized by the liver where it is hydroxylated, conjugated, and excreted in the bile. Partial reabsorption occurs and metabolic products of warfarin are excreted in urine.

Administration of warfarin. Treatment should be started with 10 mg warfarin once daily for three days. A large initial dose such as 30–40 mg is avoided as it may cause dangerous bleeding due to a rapid fall in factor VII without protecting the patient from thrombosis. Very small initial doses (2–5 mg daily) are sufficient for adequate anticoagulation in the very old, those on parenteral nutrition or recovering from cardiac surgery. The maintenance dose of warfarin varies between 1 and 20 mg daily but is usually between 3 and 8 mg. It is determined on the basis of prothrombin time ratio, which should be between 1·8 and 3·0 using the British Comparative Ratio, or between 6–11 per cent with Thrombotest. Minor surgical interventions and dental extractions can be carried out in patients whose prothrombin time ratio is below 2·5. When it is decided to cease anticoagulant treatment warfarin can be stopped and there is no need to tail it off gradually.

Change in responsiveness to warfarin. Many drugs interact with warfarin. Some that potentiate its anticoagulant effect like phenylbutazone, aspirin, indomethacin, acidic sulphonamides and anabolic steroids, act by *displacing warfarin from its albumin binding sites.* Mineral oils in laxatives, cholestyramine and broad spectrum antibiotics *reduce the availability of vitamin K* in the gastrointestinal tract, and chloramphenicol, alcohol and nortryptiline *suppress the liver enzymes that metabolize it.* Phenytoin and salicylates directly *suppress the synthesis of vitamin K-dependent factors* and thus increase a patient's sensitivity to warfarin. Increased responsiveness to oral anticoagulants is also found in infection, liver disease, hyperthyroidism and congestive cardiac failure, as well as in diarrhoea and in patients on parenteral nutrition, who develop vitamin K lack quite quickly because body stores are very small.

Barbiturates, spironolactone and glutethimide *induce liver enzymes and cause rapid metabolism of warfarin.* This results in decreased responsiveness. Thiazide diuretics and oral contraceptives also make patients resistant to warfarin. Decreased responsiveness is found in pregnancy and in lactating women. Hereditary resistance to oral anticoagulants has also been described in two large families.

Contraindications to anticoagulant treatment. Patients who have a haemorrhagic tendency, have undergone recent surgery involving the central nervous system, have a diastolic blood pressure over 110 mm Hg, have gastrointestinal lesions liable to bleed such as peptic ulcer or oesophageal varices, or have liver disease are not suitable for anticoagulant treatment.

Relative contraindications are patients who are unable or unwilling to cooperate, patients who have moderate hypertension, a previous history of peptic ulcer and renal disease. The list of contra-indications is by no means complete, and each patient must be assessed individually.

Laboratory control of oral anticoagulants. The purpose of laboratory control is to maintain stable blood concentrations of factor II, VII, IX and X at levels where thrombosis does not occur, yet the risk from bleeding is as small as possible. The test used in control is the prothrombin time. This consists in measuring the time it takes plasma to clot in the presence of thromboplastin and calcium. The therapeutic range depends entirely on the method and thromboplastin used. The results are usually expressed as a prothrombin time ratio—the ratio of patient's plasma clotting time to normal plasma clotting time. Many different thromboplastins, each giving a different therapeutic ratio are available. In the United Kingdom, human brain thromboplastin is available from the National Anticoagulant Control Reference Laboratory, in Manchester. This reagent is used as such in many laboratories or the local reagent calibrated against it.

A prothrombin time ratio obtained using the British Comparative Thromboplastin (as this reagent is called) is the British Comparative Ratio and the therapeutic range is then between *1·8 and 3·0*. This range is not absolute as some patients may require a higher ratio to prevent recurrent attacks of venous thrombosis, whereas others may bleed as soon as the ratio is above 2·0.

Another commonly used reagent is Thrombotest, a preparation containing bovine brain thromboplastin, absorbed bovine plasma, cephalin and calcium. As it already contains fibrinogen and factor V, it is not affected by changes in these factors. Clotting time is recorded as percent activity read off a graph supplied by the manufacturers. The therapeutic range is between 6–11 per cent, although patients with relative contraindications should be maintained at about 10–15 per cent.

The anticoagulant clinic. When the patient is in hospital the prothrombin time measured three times weekly during the induction period is sufficient to establish the desired therapeutic range. When the patient leaves hospital, control is best achieved through regular attendance at an anticoagulant clinic where the dose of warfarin is changed as necessary. The advantages of an anticoagulant clinic is that supervision is in the hands of personnel experienced in the field.

Patients should carry a card, which includes details of the patient, his doctor and treatment.

Complications of warfarin treatment. The commonest complications are bleeding. It is not uncommon for a patient to have repeated minor bleeds while well within the therapeutic range. The dose of warfarin in these patients must be adjusted to reduce the incidence of troublesome bleeding. Massive gastrointestinal bleeding due to an unsuspected peptic ulcer and cerebrovascular haemorrhage are the most serious complications. Apart from occasional skin rashes and diarrhoea, other complications (such as haemorrhagic skin necrosis or 'purple toe' syndrome) are extremely rare with warfarin. Agranulocytosis, renal and liver damage and exfoliative dermatitis have been reported with phenindione.

Abnormally long prothrombin ratio. This may be due to an overdose of warfarin, administration of drugs that potentiate the effects of warfarin, intercurrent infection, liver disease, renal disease or cardiac failure. A careful clinical history and examination is required to determine which of these factors are responsible.

If a patient has high prothrombin ratio without any haemorrhage it is usually enough to stop warfarin for 24–72 hours and restart with a smaller dose. If the ratio is very high (over 8·0) the patient should be observed carefully and a unit of fresh frozen plasma given to minimize the risk from the possible cerebrovascular accident or other serious haemorrhage. If the patient is bleeding, warfarin should be stopped and the patient given one to two units of plasma and blood if required. Four hours after the infusion of plasma the prothrombin time is repeated and if the ratio is still in excess of 6·0 another one to two units of plasma are given. Vitamin K_1 should not be given to patients in whom anticoagulants are to be continued, as not only does vitamin K_1 (even if given intravenously) take up to six hours to act, but it renders the patient resistant to anticoagulant treatment for some weeks. The indications for vitamin K_1 (10–20mg) i.v. or i.m. given in addition to plasma are a suicidal overdose of warfarin, suspected cerebral bleeding and bleeding in a patient who does not require further anticoagulation. Some patients in cardiac failure cannot tolerate infusion of plasma and small doses (10mg) of vitamin K_1 can be given i.v. or orally.

When drugs known to interact with warfarin are given, the prothrombin time should be taken every day or every second day during the following 7–10 days. The warfarin dose is then reduced or increased according to the prothrombin ratio. Similarly when the drug is discontinued regular prothrombin times must also be carried out during the first week.

Heparin

Heparin is a naturally occurring anionic mucopolysaccharide produced by the microsomal fraction of mast cells and basophils in all tissues. Commercially it is obtained from bovine or porcine lung or intestine. It is a white powder containing molecules of varying length and the MW varies from 9000 to 15 000. Heparin is available as the sodium or calcium salt. Each batch is different and the specific activity varies from about 110–180 iu/mg. Because of this variation, the dose of heparin is calculated in units and not in mg.

Mode of action and metabolism. When administered subcutaneously or intravenously heparin has multiple effects due to its binding and complexing with many different positively charged proteins and cations. Heparin forms a complex with a plasma protein variously called antithrombin III, anti Xa or heparin co-factor. Although this protein can neutralize thrombin in the absence of heparin, the effect is slow and incomplete. In the presence of very small doses of heparin this protein shows a marked *anti-Xa effect* (neutralization of active factor X). In the presence of higher concentrations of heparin the antithrombin effect is immediate so that the thrombin is neutralized before it can split fibrinopeptides A and B from fibrinogen. Blood is thus rendered incoagulable.

Heparin is split and inactivated in the gastrointestinal tract and hence is given parenterally. It acts immediately when given intravenously with a plasma half life of about $1\frac{1}{2}$ hours, being rapidly desulphated in the liver. Smooth anticoagulation with heparin is achieved by continuous infusion in saline or dextrose, preferably with a constant-infusion pump. Intermittent dosage involves initially excessive impairment of haemostasis with inadequate effects four hours after injection. Heparin is released slowly after subcutaneous injection and adequate levels can be maintained for 8 to 12 hours.

Administration of heparin

Prophylaxis. For prevention of venous thrombosis heparin is given subcutaneously in a dose of 5000 iu every 8 to 12 hours. The first injection is given two hours before operation and the treatment continued for 7–14 days or until the patient is fully mobile.

Treatment of thrombosis requires higher plasma levels of heparin. Treatment is started with 5000 iu intravenously followed by 25 iu per kg body weight per hour. Similar plasma levels may be achieved with subcutaneous injections of 15 000 to 20 000 iu twice daily. Warfarin is started in the three final days of heparin therapy. In calf vein thrombosis where heparin is given for three days only, the first dose of warfarin is given at the start of heparin treatment.

Contraindications to heparin treatment are similar to those for warfarin. Even conventional doses of heparin are likely to cause bleeding if given within 48 hours of major surgery or within 24 hours of childbirth. The elderly and those with impaired renal function may be unduly sensitive to heparin.

Laboratory control of heparin treatment. Five tests are commonly used for control of heparin levels (Table 22.2).

Table 22.2   Tests used in control of heparin treatment

Test	Accepted therapeutic range
Whole blood clotting time	15–25 mins.
Activated partial thromboplastin time	20–30 sec. longer than control
Calcium thrombin time	25–100 sec.*
Anti Xa assay	0·5–1·5 iu/ml
Protamine neutralization test	0·5–1·5 iu/ml

*Control 10–15 sec.

The whole blood clotting time is used most commonly but the last test is the most reliable. All tests are unreliable in patients with renal impairment or those being treated for disseminated intravascular clotting, where patients may bleed even when heparin levels are well within the therapeutic range.

The control of subcutaneously administered heparin depends on the dose used. If large doses are given the same tests as for intravenously administered heparin can be used. Laboratory control of low dose heparin (5000 iu bd or tds) for prophylaxis of venous thrombosis is rarely needed, except in patients with low platelet count or an impaired haemostatic mechanism. Under these circumstances the only available test for measuring such low levels of heparin (0·05–0·20 iu per mil) is the anti-Xa assay. Partial thromboplastin time can be used to check that excess heparin is not present in plasma. Two to three hours after subcutaneous injection patient's partial thromboplastin time should not exceed that of the control by more than 6 seconds.

Complications of heparin treatment. Haemorrhage occurs in 10 per cent of those with normal haemostasis and in almost half the patients with low platelets or with uraemia. Other complications of heparin treatment are uncommon. These are thrombocytopenia, alopecia (4–12 weeks after heparin administration), local hypersensitivity (skin necrosis at the site of injection in patients on subcutaneous heparin), general hypersensitivity reactions, and osteoporosis (in patients on high doses for long periods of time).

Treatment of heparin overdose. Withdrawal of heparin normally suffices but protamine sulphate may be needed. Protamine sulphate, a highly cationic peptide obtained from salmon or herring sperm, is an effective antidote. One milligram of protamine usually neutralizes 100 iu of heparin, the neutralizing dose being calculated from protamine neutralization test on the patients plasma. Protamine is given slowly intravenously, as it can cause a fall in blood pressure and flushing. It is important to calculate the dose as excess protamine acts as an anticoagulant.

Ancrod (Arvin)

Ancrod is the active principle of the venom obtained from the Malayan pit viper (Angkistrodon rhodostoma). It is a proteolytic enzyme which splits off fibrinopeptide A from the Aα chain of fibrinogen. Ancrod, given as a slow infusion, defibrinates the patient. The microclots deposited are readily lysed by the patient's own fibrinolytic system, and high concentrations of fibrin-split products are found in the circulation. Two to three units of Arvin per kg of body weight are given initially over 6–8 hours. Maintenance therapy is started 12 hours later as 2 u per kg body weight i.v. every 12 hours for 7 to 14 days. Three days before the end of treatment warfarin should be started.

In most patients the response of plasma fibrinogen to ancrod is remarkably predictable, and the levels of fibrinogen fall to about 5g/l. The plasma fibrinogen takes up to three weeks to return to normal after the treatment is stopped. Fibrinogen levels should be followed to detect development of resistance to ancrod.

Bleeding is the commonest complication in ancrod therapy. A proportion of patients develop resistance to ancrod due to antibody formation, and it may be impossible to give a second course of treatment. In experimental animals ancrod impairs wound healing, so it should be used with caution after surgery. It is probably contraindicated after myocardial infarction.

If rapid reversal of ancrod effects is required, a specific antivenom together with fibrinogen infusion can be used.

Streptokinase

Mode of action and metabolism. Streptokinase is a peptide isolated from the filtrate of cultures of β haemolytic streptococci. It readily forms complexes with human plasminogen and plasmin and these complexes act as activators of free plasminogen. Plasmin so generated digests fibrin in thrombi and to a lesser extent fibrinogen in the circulation. The effect of streptokinase is immediate provided all the antibodies to streptokinase in plasma have been neutralized by the initial dose. There is an immediate fall in plasminogen and fibrinogen concentration, with transient marked shortening of euglobulin lysis time and a rise in the concentration of fibrin degradation products (FDP). Slightly elevated FDP are found throughout the course of treatment. Much of the fibrinogen remaining in plasma is also partially degraded by plasmin. The thrombin time is prolonged and a transient fall in factors VIII, V and IX accompanies the induction. The changes are shown schematically in Figure 22.3.

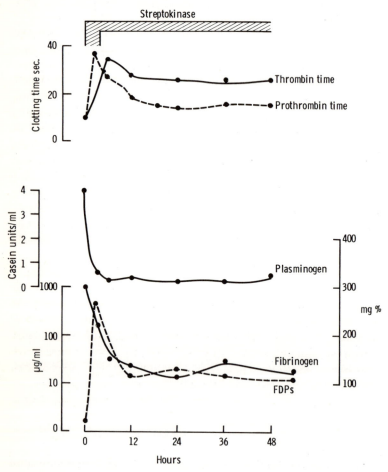

Fig. 22.3 Effect of streptokinase on laboratory tests of haemostasis.

Administration of streptokinase. Streptokinase is administered as an intravenous infusion, or in some cases of pulmonary embolism, through a catheter directly into the pulmonary artery. The initial dose is 250 000–600 000 units given to neutralize the streptococcal antibodies in the blood. As it may cause hypersensitivity reactions, the initial dose is given with 100 mg hydrocortisone i.v. The maintenance dose is 100–150 000 u hourly intravenously for 72–96 hours. Longer administration is associated with a markedly increased risk of bleeding. When the calcium thrombin time is less than twice the control time, usually four hours after stopping streptokinase, intravenous heparin should be started.

Laboratory control. Treatment is adequate when the thrombin clotting time is between 20 and 40 seconds (control 10–12 seconds). The test is first performed four hours after the initial dose and then daily for the duration of treatment. A very long thrombin time indicates hyperplasminaemia, and the dose of streptokinase should be increased to remove free plasmin. This is a difficult decision especially if the patient is bleeding and many physicians prefer to stop streptokinase infusion temporarily. A short thrombin time indicates that there is no plasmin available in the circulation because all plasminogen is complexed with streptokinase and none is available for activation and generation of plasmin. The dose of streptokinase should be reduced. The thrombin time is repeated four hours after changing the dose. Other laboratory tests which can be used in monitoring streptokinase treatment are time-consuming and include euglobulin lysis time, fibrin plate assay for activator, plasminogen assay, fibrinogen and FDP assay; if a standardized regime is used, many workers feel that no laboratory control is required.

Complications of streptokinase therapy. The main risk is bleeding. If severe, cessation of treatment with blood transfusion is preferred to the administration of antifibrinolytic agents such as epsilon-aminocaproic acid or tranexamic acid which are kept for special situations such as decision to proceed to embolectomy. EACA (100 mg/kg body weight) or tranexamic acid (10 mg/kg body weight) are given as a slow intravenous infusion. These agents are inhibitors of plasminogen activator and all clots and thrombi formed in their presence are resistant to lysis. Other untoward effects are fever and allergic reactions.

Urokinase

Urokinase is the naturally occurring plasminogen activator isolated from urine. It is an enzyme which readily cleaves plasminogen into plasmin. It is not antigenic and has a greater affinity for plasminogen in thrombi than for circulating plasminogen. Thus there are fewer haemorrhagic complications. Unfortunately it is extremely expensive.

Drugs that enhance fibrinolysis

Many substances cause the release of plasminogen activator from venous and capillary endothelium but have this effect for only a relatively short period of time. The exceptions are the combination of phenformin (a biguanide) (100 mg daily), with ethyloestranol (an anabolic steroid) (8 mg daily), and Stanozolol, which is also an anabolic steroid, given in a dose of 10 mg daily. These drugs cause a persistent increase in plasminogen activator with subsequent fall in plasma fibrinogen levels, reduction of platelet adhesion to glass beads and lowering of serum cholesterol. They may cause occasional nausea, vomiting or fluid retention and take up to three weeks to achieve the increase in fibrinolytic activity. Some encouraging results have been reported in patients with recurrent deep venous thrombosis, as well as in patients with ischaemic heart disease.

Antiplatelet drugs

Many drugs alter platelet function *in vivo* and *in vitro*, but only a few have a potential clinical use. There are: aspirin (usual dose 300–600 mg daily) which inhibits prostaglandin synthesis in the platelets, dipyridamole (100–400 mg daily) which inhibits platelet phosphodiesterase, and sulphinpyrazone (800 mg daily) whose mechanism of antiplatelet action remains unclear.

Antiplatelet drugs have been used with some success in *transient ischaemic* attacks, in particular those involving the carotid artery, in patients with prosthetic heart valves in conjunction with warfarin, in purple toe syndrome of polycythaemia rubra vera and thrombocythaemia, and in other disorders.

The drugs currently in use for their antiplatelet effects are aspirin (300–1200 mg/daily) dipyridamole (100–400 mg/day) and congeners, and sulphinpyrazone (800 mg/day).

References

Breckenridge A 1978 Oral anticoagulant drugs: Pharmacokinetic aspects. Seminars in Haematology 15: 19–26

Brozović M 1978 Oral anticoagulants in clinic practice. Seminars in Haematology 15: 27–34

Didisheim P, Fuster V 1978 Action and clinical status of platelet suppressive agents. Seminars in Haematology 15: 55–72

Nilsson I M 1974 Haemorrhagic and Thrombotic Diseases. John Wiley and Sons, New York
Pitney W R 1972 Clinical Aspects of Thrombo-embolism. Churchill Livingstone, Edinburgh
Suttie J W 1977 Oral anticoagulant therapy: the biosynthetic base. Seminars in Haematology 14: 365–374
Thomas D P 1978 Heparin in prophylaxis and treatment of venous thromboembolism. Seminars in Haematology 15: 1–18

23

Problems in the transfusion of blood

Blood transfusion involves the provision of safe and compatible blood which will have a normal survival in the patient.

The blood donor

Healthy non-anaemic adults are acceptable as donors. Pregnant women should not donate blood. Nor should persons over the age of 65 since coincidental illness may then be ascribed to the donation. People are not normally accepted as donors if they have had jaundice, malaria, a history of major allergy or recent illness. Donation of blood at six monthly intervals normally will not lead to anaemia.

Problems that may arise in the course of bleeding a donor include local bruising of the arm. Young people occasionally feel faint on standing up. If this has happened before they should rest at least 15 minutes after the donation.

A rare complication in giving blood is air embolism due to blockage of the air inlet in the bottle receiving the blood. The blood will continue to run into the bottle until the pressure in the bottle equals the raised venous pressure produced by the cuff on the donor arm. If the cuff is now released lowering the venous pressure, the flow will be from the bottle back to the donor and this will suck in a variable amount of air. This complication does not occur if blood is collected into a closed system such as plastic bags.

The blood

Normally 420 ml of blood is taken into anticoagulant which is either citrate-phosphate dextrose (CPD, anhydrous citric acid 0·21 g, anhydrous trisodium citrate 1·7 g, dextrose 1·5 g, sodium acid phosphate 0·16 g, water to 63 ml), or acid-citrate dextrose (ACD, disodium hydrogen citrate 1·7 g, dextrose 1·7 g, water to 75 ml). The enzyme 2–3 diphosphoglycerate is better preserved in CPD than ACD and hence delivery of oxygen by cells stored in CPD is better than those stored in ACD. Generally blood is preserved for up to 21 days without excessive loss of viability with both anticoagulants.

Each bottle of blood is tested serologically for the presence of hepatitis-associated antigen and for syphilis before issue. The ABO and Rhesus (D) group is re-checked. All bottles labelled Rhesus negative are of the cde/cde genotype. The serum is tested for atypical antibodies and the serum of group O donors for anti-A or B haemolysins.

Blood grouping
Some of the situations that may appear in reading results of grouping tests are shown in Table 23.1.

Compatibility testing
When patients are blood grouped their sera should also be screened for atypical antibodies against an appropriate red cell pool at the same time. For transfusion, blood of the same ABO and Rh group is selected. The red blood cells from each donor unit are tested against the patient's serum (major cross match). Because donor sera are already screened, testing of donor plasma against patient's red cells (minor cross match) is not usually carried out. The latter would normally detect dangerous Group O donors or other unusual antibody in donor serum. The cross match usually includes the following tests. In each test the donor's red cells are incubated with the recipient's serum.

1. *Saline at room temperature* to detect most cold auto- and alloantibodies, and particularly to check ABO errors.
2. *Saline at 30° C.* When apparatus is available, this technique will detect any clinically significant cold antibodies since an antibody active at 30°C may cause cell destruction *in vivo*.
3. *Saline at 37°C* to detect complete warm antibodies, and any cold antibodies with a wide thermal range.
4. *Albumin addition at 37°C* to detect incomplete warm antibodies. This may be omitted in favour of an enzyme technique.
5. *An enzyme technique* to detect incomplete warm antibodies. This is particularly sensitive for antibodies in the Rhesus system. It will not however detect all immune antibodies, and the presence of enzyme auto-antibodies of no clinical significance may confuse the result.
6. *The indirect antiglobulin technique.* This is also performed at 37°C and is the most sensitive technique available. The antiglobulin

reagent used to read the test must have a broad spectrum specificity, and be capable of detecting both IgG and complement components on the cell surface. This technique is particularly sensitive using a low ionic strength saline solution.

Under normal circumstances the tests are incubated for one hour. *Urgent provision of blood.* When blood is required under emergency conditions, the same tests as above are carried out with reduced incubation time. This however should not be less than 15 minutes. The sensitivity of the test will be increased by centrifuging the incubation mixtures at 1000 rpm for one minute, resuspending the cells and reading in the usual way. The majority of clinically significant antibodies will be detected by these methods. A full crossmatch should follow the emergency tests as it may be possible to substitute a compatible unit of blood for one issued in an emergency which has proved incompatible on more adequate testing. It is unwise to issue any blood without a compatibility test. If uncrossmatched blood is essential, it is given on the responsibility of the clinician in charge of the patient. It is possible to group a patient within minutes and hence the blood selected should be of the same ABO and Rhesus group as the patient. The use of O Rhesus Negative blood should be limited to the extremely rare cases where there is not even time to group the patient.

Patients requiring repeated transfusion. Patients who may have to be maintained on a transfusion regime for years such as those with aplastic anaemia, and other forms of marrow failure, should be fully genotyped. This information may assist in identifying atypical antibodies which may appear following multiple transfusions. It may be desirable to exclude blood with potent antigens such as Kell positive blood in Kell negative patients.

Early antibodies formed in such patients may be recognized for the first time following a transfusion and appear on the transfused red cells after 48 hours having been absent from the serum. Thus a new serum sample must always be obtained when further blood is needed since serum 48 hours later may have new antibodies. Nor should any blood remaining unused 48 hours after the initial transfusion has been given, be used unless the compatibility testing is repeated with fresh serum. Antibody coating of transfused blood can be checked by carrying out a direct antiglobulin reaction.

Transfusions in the newborn. In the newborn any antibodies present are those derived from the mother and hence cross matching of blood is done using the mother's serum.

Table 23.1 Some unexpected results from ABO grouping

Anti-A	Anti-B	Anti-A+B	Own Cells + Serum	A_1 Cells	A_2 Cells	B Cells	O Cells	
−	−	−	−	−	−	−	−	Absence of the expected antibodies. Typical of cord blood and infants under six months, agamma-globulinaemia, hypogammaglobulinaemia or sometimes in extreme age.
+++	−	+++	−	−	−	−	−	
−	+++	+++	−	−	−	−	−	
+++	+++	+++	−	−	−	−	−	
+++	−	+++	−	++	−	+++	−	A_2 with anti A_1
++	+++	+++	−	++	−	−	−	A_2B with anti A_1
±	−	±	−	+	−	+++	−	A_3 with anti A_1
−	−	++	−	+	−	+++	−	A_x with anti A_1
+++	++	+++	−	−	−	++	−	A_1 with acquired B antigen. Seen in some colonic neoplasms.
−	−	−	−	+++	+++	+++	+++	Correct cell grouping, confused by specfic cold antibodies reacting with some or all of the test cells.
+++	−	+++	−	−	+++	+++	+++	
−	+++	+++	−	+++	+++	−	+++	
+++	+++	+++	−	−	−	+++	+++	
−	−	−	+++	+++	+++	+++	+++	Correct cell groups. Serum groups complicated by an auto-antibody. Seen in autoimmune haemolytic anaemia, with cold agglutinins, with gross rouleaux after high molecular weight dextran or in myeloma.
+++	−	++	+++	+++	+++	+++	+++	
−	+++	+++	+++	+++	+++	+++	+++	
−	−	−		+++	+++	+++	+++	Oh 'Bombay' blood

Table 23.1 (continued)

Anti-A	Anti-B	Anti-A+B	Own Cells + Serum	A₁ Cells	A₂ Cells	B Cells	O Cells	
+++	+++	+++	+++	+++	+++	+++	+++	Panagglutination. This may occur in autoimmune haemolytic anaemia, gross rouleaux, severe infection, Wharton's jelly contamination of cord blood. Washing the cells with saline at 37°C may give the correct cell group.
±	±	—	±	—	—	+++	—	Dual population of cells. This is seen in rare chimera. Also due to transfusion of a different group or in a feto-maternal bleed.

Difficulties in compatibility testing

Compatibility testing is not a difficult technical procedure. Nevertheless incompatible blood is still transfused from time to time with attendant risks to the patients and on occasion a fatal outcome.

Correct working conditions. Quiet and uninterrupted working conditions are necessary. A laboratory clerk should deal with visitors and telephone calls. Interruptions increase the chance of error. Proper time must be allowed for the procurement and cross matching of blood for planned surgical admissions.

The patient's sample. Correct and proper identification of the blood sample from the patient is essential. This should include surname, first names, the hospital number, and possibly date of birth. The name alone is not adequate, as two Smiths, Jones or Patels with identical first names may be in the same ward. An unidentified emergency patient may at first be identified by number alone. The blood sample without anticoagulant should be taken by a person familiar with the patient. All samples should be re-grouped. This not only acts as a further check but checks on earlier errors in grouping whether technical or clerical. Anticoagulants are anticomplementary and samples left at room temperature tend to lose complement. These are not satisfactory for cross-matching. Samples from patients with coagulation defects will not clot properly. Fibrin strands may be removed from the tubes with sticks leaving serum and cells behind during incubation.

Reading the cross match

Rouleaux formation may confuse the results of compatibility testing in patients with myeloma, or who have been transfused a macromolecular solution. Since low molecular weight Dextran 40 has replaced high molecular weight Dextran 150, these are complications only in the enzyme techniques. Simple rouleaux is easily detected microscopically as the red cells look like piles of coins. Marked rouleaux is difficult to differentiate from agglutination, and may mask agglutination. Characteristically, rouleaux is reduced by the addition of an equal volume of saline. An appropriate control is provided by treating the patient's washed cells in the same way as donor cells. The results of the compatibility tests on each donor unit are compared with this control. The indirect antiglobulin test is unaffected.

Over exposure of cells to enzyme may give false positive reactions in the enzyme tecnique. A control of inert AB serum with the modified cells should help to interpret the reaction.

Bacterial contamination of reagents, patient's serum or donor cells may result in exposure of the T receptors of the red cell surface, giving false positive results.

The antiglobulin test although the most sensitive test available, is prone to contamination by free globulin. A scrupulously clean technique is required, and controls of both reagent and technique.

When the result is incompatible:

		SRT	S37	A/A	ENZ	IAT
Test	Donor's cells *vs* patient's serum	+ + +	—	—	—	—
Control	Patient's cells *vs* patient's serum	+ + +	—	—		—

SRT = saline at room temperature
S37 = saline at 37°C
A/A = addition of bovine albumin at 37°C
ENZ = Löws papain enzyme technique at 37°C
IAT = indirect antiglobulin test

There is a reaction between patient's serum and donor's cells at room temperature. Since this antibody agglutinates the patient's own cells to the same strength, this is a cold autoantibody. Agglutination with several donor units can be compared with the patient's own cells. Those reacting to the same degree or to a lesser degree than the patient's own cells can be used. The thermal range of the antibody is determined as those active above 30°C can cause haemolysis. Under these circumstances the direct antiglobulin test will also be positive. It should be confirmed that the antibody is Anti I (it will not react with cord blood cells). If it is active at 30°C as in cold auto-immune haemolytic anaemia the blood is warmed and transfused slowly.

		SRT	S37	A/A	ENZ	IAT
Test	Donor's cells *vs* patient's serum	+ + +	—	—	—	—
Control	Patient's cells *vs* patient's serum	—	—	—	—	—

These results denote a cold specific antibody. The specificity may include antibodies to A, A_1, B, HI, Le^a, Le^b, Lu^a, P_1, M, N or Sd^a. The specificity of the antibody may be identified by testing this patient's serum against a panel of fully genotyped cells. Blood lacking the appropriate antigen can be selected using a grouping serum, and then normal compatibility tests carried out.

		SRT	S37	A/A	ENZ	IAT
Test	Donor's cells *vs* patient's serum	—	+	+ +	+ + +	+ + +
Control	Patient's cells *vs* patient's serum	—	—	—	—	

The antibody present is a warm specific antibody with both 'complete' IgM activity in saline at 37°C and 'incomplete' IgG activity shown by the stronger reactions in albumin, enzyme and indirect antiglobulin techniques. The antibody or antibodies must be identified using a panel of cells of known genotypes. Donor blood lacking the antigen(s) is next selected using grouping sera, followed by standard compatibility tests. Antibodies giving these results could include Ss and the Rhesus system C, c, C^w, D, E or e.

		SRT	S37	A/A	ENZ	IAT
Test	Donor's cells *vs* patient's serum	—	—	—	+ +	—
Control	Patient's cells *vs* patient's serum	—	—	—	+ +	—

A disadvantage of the enzyme technique is the occasional enzyme auto-antibody. This is usually of no importance provided that the reaction of the donor's cells is the same strength or weaker than that of the patient's cells. Alternatively these results could be due to overexposure of the cells to enzyme. The enzyme-treated cell control (using AB serum to replace patient's serum) if negative will indicate that over-modification is not the cause of this reaction. These results would also be obtained if low molecular weight Dextran had been given to the patient before the blood sample was taken. If there is no serum available prior to Dextran infusion, it may be possible to disperse the rouleaux with addition of an equal volume of saline. Reliance is placed on the direct antiglobulin result.

		SRT	S37	A/A	ENZ	IAT
Test	Donor's cells *vs* patient's serum	—	—	—	+ +	—
Control	Patient's cells *vs* patient' serum	—	—	—	—	—

If there is a reaction using the enzyme technique with donor's cells and not patient's cells, a specific antibody is present. The enzyme technique is very sensitive and may detect antibodies, particularly of the Rhesus system, before they are detected by any other technique. Low affinity antibodies may be present to a high titre by enzyme techniques and yet be difficult to detect using the indirect antiglobulin reaction. Nevertheless these are clinically significant. Antigens destroyed and therefore not detected by enzyme technique include M, N, S, Fy^a, and Fy^b. The specific enzyme antibody is identified using the enzyme technique and a panel of genotyped cells. Donor blood is selected which lacks the antigen, and normal compatibility procedures are carried out.

		SRT	S37	A/A	ENZ	IAT
Test	Donor's cells *vs* patient's serum	—	—	—	—	+ + +
Control	Patient's cells *vs* patient's serum	—	—	—	—	—

The antibodies in some blood group systems are only identified by the antiglobulin technique. These include Kell, Duffy and Kidd. Lewis antibodies bind complement and are detected using an antiglobulin reagent which contains anti-β_1 components. The specific antibody in this example is identified using a cell panel and the indirect antiglobulin technique. Blood lacking the antigen is selected using grouping serum, and compatibility tests are performed. Occasionally a donor is found to have a positive direct direct antiglobulin test, and that one unit will therefore appear incompatible with any sera.

		SRT	S37	A/A	ENZ	IAT
Test	Donor's cells *vs* patient's serum	—	—	+ +	+ + +	+ + +
Control	Patient's cells *vs* patient's serum	—	—	+ +	+ + +	+ + +

In autoimmune haemolytic anaemia with 'warm' antibodies, the serum reacts strongly with all cell samples. Any transfused blood will have reduced cell survival. An attempt may be made to identify an underlying specificity. Serial dilutions of the patient's serum are tested against a panel of cells of differing Rhesus genotypes, –D- and Rh null cells. If there is evidence of specificity, the Rhesus genotype lacking this antigen should be given. For example, if the specificity appears to be anti-e, R_2R_2 (ccDEE) blood will be taken. Compatibility tests are carried out on several units in parallel with the patient's own cells.

The strength of agglutination by each technique is recorded, and the 'least incompatible' blood selected.

The use of blood components

Red blood cells. 'Packed' red cells are prepared by removing most of the supernatant plasma from the centrifuged blood. Its use is indicated when the need is to correct anaemia without expanding plasma volume unduly, e.g. in severe pernicious anaemia with incipient cardiac failure. Red cells are being supplied by transfusion centres to an increasing extent because the plasma is used for preparation of other blood products. Red cells relatively free of plasma, white cells and platelets are required in patients who have become sensitized to these substances and who have transfusion reactions as a result. Red cells can be washed relatively free of these components by several resuspensions in saline followed by centrifugation. The reconstitution of red cells initially preserved under liquid nitrogen provides a red cell suspension relatively free of other components and should be used in those patients in whom simple procedures have been ineffective in preventing transfusion reactions.

Platelets. Platelets concentrated from fresh plasma and kept at 22°C with constant agitation, survive as well as fresh platelets when transferred to a donor within 24 hours. There is a risk of infection in platelets stored at room temperature; even small numbers of organisms are dangerous in those patients who require platelets, e.g. patients receiving cytotoxic drugs for treatment of leukaemia, a malignant tumour or during the course of a marrow transplant. Platelets may also be required in some drug-induced thrombocytopenias and aplasias. They are of little value in autoimmune purpuras as the platelets are rapidly cleared from the circulation when antibodies are present. Nevertheless, patients with severe bleeding due to thrombocytopenia of any aetiology should be given platelets.

In the absence of abnormal sequestration, the rise in platelet count from transfusion of the platelets from one unit of blood is about $12000/\mu l$. Generally about one third of the platelets given are recovered in the recipient's plasma. Platelets from not less than five units of blood are required to obtain a significant rise in platelet count in an adult. With repeated platelet transfusions allo-antibodies against platelets appear so that progressively poorer results are obtained. Ideally platelets from donor and recipient should have not only similar ABO and Rhesus systems but also similar HL–A groups. A sibling may fulfil these conditions and under these circumstances platelets transfusions can be continued from the same donor for several years.

Neutrophils. Meaningful transfusion of leucocytes is only possible when a special cell separator is available that enables one to recirculate a donor's blood through the machine and in this way harvest relatively large amounts of leucocytes or other component such as platelets. Although the half time of neutrophils in the blood is only 6–7 hours with a longer survival in the tissues, white cell transfusion may prove useful in overcoming intractable infection in patients e.g. with leukaemia receiving cytotoxic drugs. White cells have also been transfused as a source of a source of 'transfer factor'.

Plasma. Plasma is available as a plasma protein fraction which contains albumin and heat stable alpha-and-beta globulins prepared from a large pool of human plasma. It is stored as a clear liquid and has a two year shelf life. It does not contain isoagglutinins and can be given regardless of blood group. Although a large pool of plasma is involved, the hepatitis risk is minimal due to prolonged incubation at 60°C. Plasma protein fraction is used as a volume expander. Fresh plasma (stored in the frozen state) and cryoprecipitate are discussed in Chapter 16. Albumin and gamma-globulin concentrates are also prepared.

Untoward transfusion reactions

Immediate transfusion reactions

A patient having a severe transfusion reaction complains of low back pain, fever, shivering, sensation of tightness in the chest, nausea and vomiting. There is a rapid pulse rate and a fall of blood pressure. This may be followed by abnormal bleeding, reduced output of urine and even complete anuria. These are the symptoms of a haemolytic transfusion reaction. Another type of reaction occurring during transfusion is the development of fever sometimes with shivering. This can be due to sensitivity to leucocytes, platelets, plasma or rarely nowadays to pyrogens but also to extravascular destruction of incompatible red cells.

A third type of reaction to blood is the appearance of itching and wheals (urticaria) sometimes with tightness of the chest (broncho-spasm). This allergic reaction is usually due to sensitivity to plasma components.

Delayed transfusion reactions

Here there are none of the symptoms described above. Nevertheless the patient does not benefit from the transfusion and haemoglobin either fails to rise or the rise is shortlived. There may be jaundice. This is due to a secondary immune response in which the transfused blood is eliminated. Post-transfusion purpura has been described in Chapter 14.

Other untoward results

Despite screening of bloods for hepatitis-associated antigen, serum hepatitis and jaundice remain a risk. The time elapsing between the transfusion and the appearance of jaundice is 60–160 days, although rarely it may be shorter. It is far more likely to occur in patients receiving large numbers of blood units.

Cytomegalic virus infection with a glandular fever-like blood picture may occur in patients undergoing by-pass surgery and in whom more than 20 units of blood are used for transfusion and priming of the equipment. Malaria has also been transmitted by transfusion of blood.

Transfusion of blood contaminated by bacteria gives rise to profound shock, fever, rigor, pains, and drop in blood pressure. The mortality is high.

Overtransfusion, particularly in anaemic patients with poor cardiac function, leads to an excessive blood volume, cardiac failure and pulmonary oedema. The earliest sign is a repeated cough and examination shows moist sounds in the chest. This is followed by marked dyspnoea and raised jugular venous pressure. The symptoms often come on 24 hours after the transfusion. Patients at risk should be transfused cautiously with packed red cells accompanied by a diuretic. When signs of overload appear a further diuretic should be given and, if necessary, a venesection is carried out.

In the long term immunization of the recipient to red cell and tissue antigens may occur. Repeated transfusion leads to marked accumulation of iron in the body and a clinical picture of haemosiderosis.

Transfusion of many units of blood over a short period may introduce problems of citrate toxicity. This anticoagulant does not normally affect adults but in infants, especially following exchange transfusion, may cause a fall in plasma calcium. To prevent this, heparin is added to the blood, followed by calcium gluconate. Individuals with liver disease may have impaired citrate metabolism, and show a depression of ionised calcium. Transfusion of large volumes of stored blood may dilute coagulation factors V and VIII and reduce the platelet count. This may potentiate bleeding. Fresh plasma is given if the coagulation screen shows depletion of clotting factors. It is rarely necessary to give platelets.

Rapid transfusion of refrigerated blood may lower the temperature of the patient and can cause cardiac irregularity. Blood may be given through a blood warmer, maintained at 37°C.

Management and investigation of a transfusion reaction

As soon as a transfusion reaction is recognized, the transfusion of the blood is stopped and saline substituted. If necessary steps are taken to combat shock and maintain renal function.

The first action must be to determine whether or not a haemolytic reaction has occurred. A blood sample is collected with care to avoid haemolysis, and the plasma is examined. Comparison with a pretransfusion sample will show free haemoglobin (a pink colour) or methaemalbumen (a brown colour) in the presence of significant haemolysis. This is particularly important in a bleeding patient who may need blood urgently. At the same time checks for a clerical error are instituted within the laboratory, the ward and/or operating theatre.

If a haemolytic transfusion reaction has occurred, a fluid output chart is started. All urine passed is retained. Twenty g of mannitol in 100 ml is given intravenously and this can be repeated if diuresis does not follow until it is clear that renal tubular necrosis has occurred. Thereafter the appropriate regime is instituted until there is regeneration of the renal tubules. If there is evidence of disseminated intravascular coagulation appropriate replacement therapy may be required. Shock is treated by warmth and by maintaining blood pressure by giving compatible blood when this is available.

If no clerical error has occurred, and this includes collection of the initial blood sample from the correct patient, correct labelling in ward and of tubes in the laboratory, exclusion of mix-up in labelling of donor units or simply blood labelled for one patient given in error to another, further investigations are instituted. The following samples must be obtained:

1. Pretransfusion sample of the patients blood.
2. The donor blood samples used for crossmatching.
3. The residue of the offending unit of blood and other units already transfused.
4. A heparinized and EDTA post-transfusion sample from the patient.
5. A clotted post-transfusion sample from the patient.
6. Urine passed during and after the transfusion.

1. and 2. will be available in a properly managed laboratory and 3.

must be retrieved from the ward or theatre; 4. and 5. are collected from the patients arm not being used for transfusion with a wide-bore needle, disposable syringe and without any spirits on the arm.

Culture for bacterial contamination of the unit of blood is set up as soon as possible. This is exceedingly rare and to the naked eye such blood may be haemolyzed with clots and purplish in colour. The commonest organisms are pseudomonas and coliforms. Examination of a gram stained blood film from the bottle may show organisms. A haemolysed donor unit in the absence of bacterial contamination may result from overheating or inadvertant freezing and thawing of the blood. Overheating will produce damaged red cells visible in a blood film. The practice of adding drugs to the blood unit can damage red cells and this includes diuretics such as ethacrynic acid.

Table 23.2   Investigation of a transfusion reaction.

When the reaction is notified	Obtain a full account of the circumstances of this reaction. Obtain the blood unit. Take 10 ml clotted blood. Take 5 ml EDTA and 5 ml heparinised blood. Take the first urine passed. Start a fluid intake chart. Check all clerical records. Find the pretransfusion sample and the red cell suspension prepared from donor blood.
Unit of blood	Check the labelling, group, expiry date and name label. Check the general appearance. Blood culture. Gram stain. ABO group and Rh type. Screen for atypical antibodies.
Heparin blood	Examine the plasma for haemolysis.
Pre-transfusion sample	ABO group and Rh type. Screen for atypical antibodies. Repeat compatibility tests.
Post-transfusion sample	Examine the serum for evidence of haemolysis or jaundice. ABO group and Rh type. Screen for atypical antibodies. Repeat compatibility tests. Direct antiglobulin test. Examine red cells microscopically for clumping. Test the serum for methaemalbumin, haptoglobins and bilirubin.
Urine	Test for haemoglobin, urobilinogen and haemosiderin. Examine microscopically for red cells.
EDTA sample	Full blood count and film.

Thereafter further tests are performed for haemoglobin products in serum and urine. In addition to discoloration of heparinized plasma (light pink with free haemoglobin of 20 mg/100 ml) smaller amounts can be detected with a spectroscope. The maximum bilirubin level is reached between 3–8 hours (jaundiced plasma). After four hours methaemalbumin is looked for by Schumm's test. The urine is examined for free haemoglobin and pigments. Red cells from the post-transfusion blood sample are resuspended in saline and examined for agglutinates. These may be present after an ABO incompatible transfusion. Thereafter all the blood samples listed above are re-grouped. Steps are taken to detect weak groups of A in the donor blood. Absence of the expected anti-A or anti-B in the patient's post-transfusion serum may indicate ABO incompatible transfusion. A marked increase in titre of agglutinins in these cases occurs in the second week. A mixed-field appearance in the post-transfusion sample in agglutination tests may be present, either agglutinated A cells in an O recipient or agglutinated Rh positive cells in an Rh negative recipient.

The direct antiglobulin test is carried out on the pre- and post-transfusion samples. A negative pre-transfusion test that has become positive suggests that the donor cells were incompatible with the patient's serum. Finally the cross-matches are set up again against both pre- and post-transfusion serum samples. Any antibodies discovered are identified. The procedures are summarized in Table 23.2.

The causes of transfusion reactions

The commonest cause is clerical error at some stage between the collection of the initial blood sample from the patient to the final error of giving a properly labelled unit of blood to the wrong patient.

Severe haemolytic transfusion reactions are most often due to ABO incompatible blood being given. This is because antibodies within this system are normally present. The reaction starts following transfusion of a few ml of blood and the effects depend on the volume of incompatible blood given. Under anaesthesia, transfusion reactions are suppressed and the patient may recover with jaundice, anuria or anaemia. Intravascular haemolysis is due to either IgM or IgG antibodies.

When the antibody is not haemolytic e.g. anti-D, the red cell destruction is largely extravascular, the sensitized cells being cleared from the circulation. The transfusion reaction may be clinically milder although fever and rigor is common and free haemoglobin may appear in plasma. Occasionally, Group O donor blood may contain an immune anti-A and/or anti-B and this can cause a haemolytic reaction when given to an A, B or AB patient. Rarely anti-D can be transfused in this way.

A delayed transfusion reaction in which the transfused blood is removed within the week following transfusion may be difficult to anticipate. Immune antibodies including anti-D may have virtually disappeared from blood or be present in such low titre as to be undetectable. This may be the situation in an Rh-negative person sensitized by a Rh-positive pregnancy. A transfusion of D-positive blood many years later may produce a secondary response with a rapid clearance of the transfused cells.

Previous pregnancies or previous transfusions may lead to the appearance of antibodies to leucocytes, platelets and serum proteins. If one is satisfied that the transfusion reaction is of this type the transfusion can be allowed to continue, hydrocortisone and anti-histaminics being given to suppress the reaction. Subsequent transfusions may require the use of washed red cells.

Index